Nancy Clark's
SPORTS NUTRITION GUIDEBOOK

Nancy Clark, MS, RD
Nutritionist
SportsMedicine Brookline
Brookline, MA

Illustrations by Bill Pardy

Leisure Press
Champaign, Illinois

Library of Congress Cataloging-in-Publication Data

Clark, Nancy, 1951-
    Nancy Clark's sports nutrition guidebook / by Nancy Clark.
        p.   cm.
    Bibliography: p.
    Includes index.
    ISBN 0-88011-326-X
    1. Athletes--Nutrition   I. Title.   II. Title: Sports nutrition
    guidebook.
    TX361.A8C54   1990
    613.2'024796--dc20   89-8179
                                                                        CIP

ISBN: 0-88011-326-X

Developmental Editor: Peggy Rupert, MA; Copyeditor: Wendy Nelson; Assistant Editors: Holly Gilly, Rob King, Timothy Ryan, Julia Anderson; Proofreader: Claire Mount; Production Director: Ernie Noa; Typesetters: Cindy Pritchard, Angela K. Snyder; Text Design: Keith Blomberg; Text Layout: Tara Welsch; Cover Design: Jack Davis; Illustrations: Bill Pardy; Printer: Versa Press

Printed in the United States of America

15   14   13   12   11   10   9

Leisure Press
A Division of Human Kinetics Publishers
Box 5076, Champaign, IL 61825-5076
1-800-747-4457

Canada: Human Kinetics Publishers P.O. Box 2503 Windsor,
ON N8Y 4S2
1-800-465-7301 (in Canada only)

Europe: Human Kinetics Publishers (Europe) Ltd. P.O. Box IW14,
Leeds LS16 6TR, England
0532-781708

Australia: Human Kinetics Publishers, P.O. Box 80,
Kingswood 5062, South Australia
618-374-0433

New Zealand: Human Kinetics Publishers, P.O. Box 105-231,
Auckland 1
(09) 309-2259

To my husband, John McGrath.
He nourishes me with his love.

Contents

Acknowledgments

With sincere thanks and appreciation to

My clients, for teaching me about sports nutrition "in the raw." Working with them has made me a more effective sports nutritionist. I have changed clients' names in this book to protect their privacy.

Cynthia Howard, a nutrition graduate student at Massachusetts General Hospital Institute of Health Professions, for being a dedicated research assistant.

Bill Pardy, for adding a touch of humor to a heavy work load.

Peggy Rupert, editor, for her good advice and assistance.

Dr. William Southmayd, medical director of SportsMedicine Systems, Inc., for his continual support.

Sue Luke, MS, RD, nutritionist at SportsMedicine Boston, for proofreading and professional assistance, as well as for being a caring friend.

My family, for their loving support.

Recipe Contributors

My special thanks go to the following food lovers who shared their special recipes. In some cases, I adjusted their ingredients to meet my criteria for easy preparation and lower fat content.

Deborah Allen, Newton, MA	Cheesecake Snackwich
Shawn Amirault, Nova Scotia	Zucchini Cake
Gabriella Andersen, Sun Valley, ID	Three-Seed Yeast Bread
Jane Balboni, N. Attleboro, MA	Maple Graham Shake
David Bastille, Holliston, MA	Pasta With Pesto
Mary Bernazanni, Boston, MA	Pizza Fondue
Joan Betterly, Sterling, MA	Cheesy Bean and Rice Casserole
Chris Brown, Concord, NH	Orange-Oatmeal Bread
Caroline Clark, N. Dartmouth, MA	Apple Brown Betty
Janice Clark, Little Compton, RI	Oatmeal Raisin Cookies, Goulash
Candace Crowell, Georgetown, MA	Blueberry Buckle
Melynda Curran, Lynnfield, MA	Beans Baked With Apples
Donna Diefenbach, Boston, MA	Chicken 'N' Cheese
Pam Duckworth, Brookline, MA	Granola
Robyn Fass, Stockton, CA	Fruit Smoothie
Bill and Dottie Fine, Boston, MA	Lazy Lasagna
Ellen Herbert, Newton, MA	Beef in Beer
Jane Houmes, Phoenix, AZ	Company Rice Salad
Cynthia Howard, Boston, MA	Pasta Salad Parmesan
R.M. Lane, National Ski Patrol	Hot Spiced Tea Mix
Sue Luke, Holliston, MA	A-To-Z Cake
Sandy and Andy Miller, Boston, MA	Hamburger-Noodle Feast
Catherine McGrath, Buffalo, NY	Irish Soda Bread

John McGrath, Waltham, MA	Chili
Emmy Norris, Billerica, MA	Banana Frostie
Elaine Price, Boston, MA	Irish Tacos
Quaker Oats Co., Barrington, IL	Cinnamon Oat Bran Muffins, Oatmeal Pancakes
Fran Richman, Boston, MA	Chicken Baked With Mustard, Tofu Salad Dressing
Dave Selsky, Boston, MA	Crunchy Fish Fillets
Diane Sinski, Belmont, MA	Stir-Fried Chicken With Apple and Curry
Jean Smith, Newton, MA	Potato Snacks, Crunchy Peanut Butter Sandwich
Susan Westin, Brockton, MA	Chocolate Lush

Foreword

Proper nutrition is essential for any athlete who seeks to attain enduring success and health. But the importance of sports nutrition has been overlooked for many years. In fact, when I became team physician for the Boston Celtics 3 years ago, I was amazed at how many of these talented athletes did not fully realize the direct relationship between proper sports nutrition and size, strength, endurance, conditioning, and injury prevention.

Nancy Clark offers a winning game plan for sports nutrition that will improve the performance potential of every athlete. Her writing style makes each topic easy to read and easy to remember. All it takes to benefit from her straightforward coaching is a little practice, determination, and discipline. It's that basic and simple.

Describing each concept in layperson's terms, Nancy explains the benefits of using natural, wholesome foods to fulfill caloric needs, to supply protein to aid strengthening and growth, and to provide basic vitamins without the use of supplements. At the same time, she dispels many myths about nutrition, including those which advocate high-fat diets.

Nancy Clark's Sports Nutrition Guidebook will also help you learn how to lose or gain weight the healthy way, discover how to best replace your body fluids, and find out how to time your meals to enhance your athletic performance. Nancy's recipes and meal menus are creative, inexpensive, and simple to make. Best of all, the food is great to eat.

There's also a chapter devoted to two of my favorite subjects, snacks and snack attacks. Let's face it, few of us survive on just three meals a day. Nancy Clark addresses the issue of snacking and provides a sensible way to handle those "irresistible" snack attacks. She also offers a strategic method for raiding the refrigerator.

Nancy Clark is a true scientist and teacher when it comes to nutrition. As a past ''protein-aholic'' and refrigerator sneak thief, I consider *Nancy Clark's Sports Nutrition Guidebook* a landmark in sports nutrition, athletic training, and sports medicine.

Arnold D. Scheller
Staff Physician, SportsMedicine Brookline
Team Physician, Boston Celtics
Clinical Assistant Professor, Department of Orthopedic Surgery
   Tufts University School of Medicine

Preface

Everyone wins with good nutrition!

"My diet is horrendous! I continually drink too much coffee. I skip lunch four out of five workdays. I raid the candy machine every afternoon. I grab dinner on the run five out of seven nights. I either have to lose weight or buy a whole new wardrobe. I know I should eat better, but I just don't make the effort to."

Perhaps this story sounds familiar to you. It's just one version of the frustrations I commonly hear expressed by my clients. This runner/lawyer felt overwhelmed by all his unfulfilled nutrition shoulds: "I know what I should eat, I just don't do it . . ." If you feel this same frustration and sense of failure, rest assured that the solution is easier than you think.

As a registered dietitian and sports nutritionist, I teach many types of sports-active people how to be successful with their eating. Together we develop a desirable sports diet that they can realistically incorporate into their schedules, based on their eating patterns, food likes and dislikes, weight goals, work and workout schedules, time constraints, and cooking skills and interests.

The purpose of *Nancy Clark's Sports Nutrition Guidebook* is to help you gain a clear perspective on food for health, fitness, sports, weight control, and fun—all in the context of an on-the-go lifestyle. You'll learn how you can thrive on healthful high-energy foods, regardless of your cooking skills or hectic schedule. You'll lose your fears that good nutrition means little more than eating tofu and bean sprouts!

When I first started working at the Boston-area SportsMedicine Brookline, one of the largest sports medicine clinics in the United States, I struggled to sell the concept that food works for you—that what you eat can enhance your sports performance. Eight years later, active people of all ages and abilities, from amateurs to Olympic champions, come to me seeking sports nutrition advice. Many of these sports-active people strive to eat top-quality diets but find it difficult to eat nutritiously with their eat-and-run lifestyles.

They want to be sure that

- their daily training diet supports their athletic aspirations,
- their precompetition meals offer the winning edge, and
- their daily food choices promote future health and longevity.

Over the years, my clients have given me invaluable insights into their nutrition misconceptions and food foibles, ''magic'' sports foods, secret pregame meals, tasty cooking tips, and steps to recovery from eating disorders. My own firsthand experiences with eating for track workouts, marathon running, cross-country bicycling, trekking, skiing, winter camping, AND eating on the run enriched my college and graduate education in nutrition and exercise physiology. In these pages I share these experiences and teach you my approach to helping

- marathon runners go the distance,
- dancers and wrestlers lose weight successfully,
- aspiring young athletes compete at their best, and
- parents provide optimal nutrition for themselves and their families.

You'll glean a concise understanding of ways to enhance your diet, as have many of the champions I've helped, including the Boston Celtics, Olympic figure skater Kitty Carruthers, professional golfer Brad Faxon, Wimbledon tennis player Tim Mayotte, and marathoner Bill Rodgers.

Contrary to popular belief, you won't have to give up the foods that taste good, commit yourself to nutrition martyrdom, or imprison yourself in the kitchen. Nor will you have to forego fast foods, drastically change your lifestyle, or deny yourself the pleasures of eating. In the following pages, you'll learn how to balance the good with the not-so-good and gradually phase into eating *more* of the best and less of the rest. You'll win by learning how to choose a daily sports diet that prepares you for tough competitions and lifelong health.

Enjoy your success!

Nancy Clark, MS, RD
SportsMedicine Brookline
830 Boylston St.
Brookline, MA 02167

SECTION I

Your Daily Training Diet

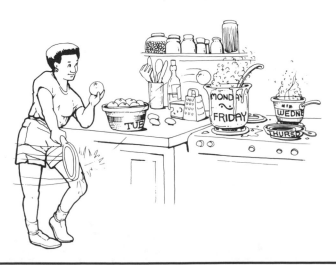

CHAPTER 1

A Game Plan
for Good Nutrition

"I know what I should eat. I just don't do it."

I hear this said every day by students, parents, business people, and athletes. They struggle with juggling work and workouts, family and friends, food and nutrition. They make time to exercise but don't always make time to eat right.

This chapter will help you design your own good nutrition game plan. Whether you're a fitness exerciser or an Olympic athlete, you can (and you know that you should) give yourself optimal nutrition with wholesome foods even if you're eating on the run. The trick is to grab the foods that both support your sports program and enhance your health.

To learn how to do this, keep reading! Knowing what is good for you doesn't necessarily mean that you will choose what is good for you, but at least you will know your options.

The Six Nutrients for Health

Food is more than just bulk that stops your hunger; it is a fuel composed of important nutrients essential for maintaining optimal health and top performance. There are six types of nutrients:

Carbohydrate

A source of calories that fuels your muscles and brain. Carbohydrates are the primary energy source when you're exercising hard. You should get 60 percent of your calories from the starches and sugars found in carbohydrate-rich foods such as fruits, vegetables, breads, and grains.

Fats

A source of stored energy (calories) that we burn primarily during low-level activity, such as reading and sleeping. Animal fats (for example, butter, lard, fat in meats) tend to be saturated and to contribute to heart disease and some cancers; vegetable fats (for example, corn oil, olive oil, peanut oil) are generally unsaturated and less harmful. You should limit your fat intake to about 25 percent of your daily total calories.

Protein

Essential for building and repairing muscles, red blood cells, hair, and other tissues, and for synthesizing hormones. Protein is digested into amino acids, which are rebuilt into the protein in muscle and other tissues. Protein is a source of calories and can be used for energy if inadequate carbohydrates are available such as during a strict diet or exhausting exercise. About 15 percent of your calories should come from protein-rich foods such as fish, chicken, and dried beans.

Vitamins

Metabolic catalysts that regulate the chemical reactions within the body. They include vitamins A, B complex, C, D, E, and K. Most vitamins are chemical substances that the body does not manufacture, so you must obtain them through your diet. They are not a source of energy (calories).

Minerals

Elements obtained from foods that combine in many ways to form structures of the body (for example, calcium in bones) and regulate body processes (for example, iron in red blood cells transports oxygen). Other important minerals are magnesium, phosphorus, sodium, potassium, and zinc. Minerals do not provide energy.

Water

An essential substance that makes up about 50 to 55 percent of your weight. Water stabilizes body temperature, carries nutrients to and waste away from cells, and is needed for cells to function. Water does not provide energy.

To help you determine whether you're getting the right balance of these nutrients, the U.S. Government has established the Recommended Dietary Allowance (RDA) as a standard for nutrient intake. The recommendations for vitamins and minerals meet or exceed the needs of nearly all people, including athletes.

In the following pages you will learn how to eat a high-energy, healthful combination of foods that provides the RDA of important nutrients and promotes your health and fitness.

The RDA Versus U.S. RDA

The Recommended *Dietary* Allowance (RDA) is not a requirement but rather an estimate of a safe and adequate nutrient intake that will maintain good health. You should try to meet the RDA on a daily basis. If your daily intake fluctuates, but your average weekly intake meets the allowances, you are unlikely to suffer from nutritional deficiencies.

The United States Recommended *Daily* Allowance (U.S. RDA) is listed on food labels and, for each nutrient listed, is a standard based on the population group with the highest RDA needs for that nutrient—most often growing teenage boys. Because women have the highest RDA for iron, the U.S. RDA is based on women's need and is overly generous for men.

Following are the U.S. RDA standards for adults and children over 4 years old:

Protein	65 g
Vitamin A	5,000 IU
Vitamin C	60 mg
Thiamin	1.5 mg
Riboflavin	1.7 mg
Niacin	20 mg
Calcium	1 g
Iron	18 mg
Vitamin D	400 IU

Three Keys to Healthful Eating

When choosing your meals and snacks, base your nutrition game plan on these three important keys to healthful eating:

1.   Variety. There is no one magic food. Each food offers special nutrients. For example, oranges provide vitamin C and carbohydrates but not iron or protein. Beef offers iron and protein but not vitamin C or carbohydrates. You'll thrive best by eating a variety of foods.

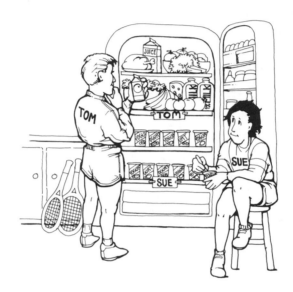

I often counsel athletes who have severely restricted their diets. One runner, for example, limited herself to plain yogurt, rice cakes, and oranges. Besides lacking variety, her diet lacked iron, zinc, and vitamins A, E, and K, and more as well.

2.   Moderation. Even soda pop and chips, in moderation, can fit into a well-balanced diet. Simply balance out refined sugars and fats with nutrient-wise choices at your next meal. For example, compensate for a greasy sausage and biscuit breakfast by selecting a low-fat turkey sandwich lunch. Although no one food is a junk food, too many nutrient-poor selections can accumulate into a junk-food diet.

3. Wholesomeness. Choose natural or lightly processed foods as often as possible: for instance, whole wheat rather than white bread, apples rather than apple juice, and baked potatoes rather than potato chips. Natural foods generally have more nutritional value and fewer questionable additives.

You don't have to eat three square meals a day to have a well-rounded diet; you only need to choose a variety of wholesome foods from the four major food groups: Dairy products, Fruits and Vegetables, Meats and Protein-alternates, Grains and Cereals.

Each type of food provides different vitamins and minerals. You store these nutrients in your body—some in stockpiles, such as the vitamin A made from the beta-carotene found in carrots, tomato sauce, and broccoli; some in smaller amounts, such as the vitamin C from orange juice, green peppers, and cantaloupe.

By wisely selecting 1,200 to 1,500 calories per day from a variety of wholesome foods, you can consume the RDA of the vitamins, minerals, amino acids, and other nutrients (other than calories) you need for good health. Because many active people consume 2,000 to 5,000 calories (depending on their age, level of activity, body size, and gender), nutrient excesses are more common among hungry athletes than are deficiencies. For example, one of my clients, a football player, guzzled 5 times the RDA of vitamin C in his mere snack of a quart of orange juice.

Unlike most hockey players, hikers, and cyclists, who usually are hearty eaters, runners, wrestlers, and gymnasts are generally weight-conscious; they often worry about fattening calories and overlook the fact that food also provides essential nutrients. These athletes need to carefully select nutrient-dense foods—foods that offer the most nutritional value for the fewest calories—to reduce the risk of a nutrient-deficient diet.

To help you select the nutrient-dense foods that fit your lifestyle, follow this good nutrition game plan.

Good Nutrition Game Plan: Dairy Products

Some best choices: low-fat milk, yogurt, and low-fat cheeses (such as part-skim mozarella, string cheese, "lite" brands of cheddar-type cheese). Minimum daily intake to obtain adequate daily calcium:

- 4 servings* (1,200 mg) for growing teens and children
- 3 servings* (800 mg) for men
- 3 or 4 servings* (800 to 1,500 mg) for women

Postmenopausal and other amenorrheic women may need 1,200 to 1,500 milligrams of calcium.

---

*One serving is equivalent to 8 ounces of milk or yogurt (preferably low-fat) or 1.5 ounces of cheese (2 average slices of American cheese).

Main nutrients: calcium, protein, riboflavin

Protective benefits:

- Maintain strong bones
- Reduce risk of osteoporosis
- Protect against high blood pressure
- Protect against muscle cramps

Make no bones about it! Low-fat milk and other calcium-rich dairy products should be an important part of your diet throughout your lifetime. Your bones are alive and need calcium on a daily basis. Children and teens need calcium for growth. Adults also need calcium to maintain strong bones. Although you may stop growing by age 20, your bones don't reach peak density until age 30 to 35. The amount of calcium stored in your bones at that age is a critical factor influencing your susceptibility to fractures as you get older. After age 35, bones start to thin as a normal part of aging. A calcium-rich diet in combination with exercise can slow this process.

The Best Sources of Calcium

Low-fat milk and yogurt made from low-fat or nonfat milk are among the richest sources of calcium. They are also among the healthiest because they have most of the fat removed. A glass of whole milk has the equivalent of two pats of butter, but skim milk has next to none.

Type of milk	% Fat by weight	% Fat by calories
Whole milk	3.5	48
2% Low-fat milk	2	38
1% Low-fat milk	1	28
Skim milk	trace	4

Although ice cream can be a fair source of calcium (2 cups of ice cream is the calcium equivalent of 1 cup of milk), it also contains excessive saturated fat and cholesterol, two risk factors related to heart disease. I suggest that ice cream be replaced with frozen yogurt or other low-fat, calcium-rich selections (see Table 1.1).

Table 1.1   Calcium, Cholesterol, and Fat in Dairy Products

Dairy Product	Amount	Calories	Fat (g)	Cholesterol (mg)	Calcium (mg)
Milk, whole	1 c	150	8	34	290
2% low-fat	1 c	120	5	18	300
1% low-fat	1 c	100	3	10	300
Skim	1 c	85	trace	4	300
Yogurt, low-fat					
plain	1 c	145	4	14	415
vanilla	1 c	195	3	11	390
fruit	1 c	240–260	3	10	315
Cheese					
American	1 oz	105	9	27	175
Cheddar	1 oz	115	10	30	200
Mozzarella, part skim	1 oz	80	5	15	205
Ricotta, part skim	1/2 c	170	10	38	340
Cottage, creamed	1/2 c	120	5	17	70
Cottage, 1% fat	1/2 c	80	1	5	70
Ice Cream					
Regular vanilla	1 c	270	14	60	180
Rich vanilla	1 c	350	24	90	150
Ice milk, vanilla	1 c	185	6	18	175
Soft-serve, Dairy Queen	med	230	7	20	200
Shake, vanilla McDonald's	lg	350	8	31	300
Safe intake					
Women		1,800–2,200+	50–60	<300	1,200
Men		2,200–3,500+	60–95	<300	800+

Note. Nutrient data from *Bowes and Church's Food Values of Portions Commonly Used* (14th ed.) by J. Pennington and H. Church, 1985, Philadelphia: Lippincott. Adapted by permission.

Dairy products are not the only sources of calcium, but they are convenient for eat-and-runners. Significant amounts of calcium are also found in the following foods:

- Dark, leafy vegetables such as broccoli, collards, and kale (however, the calcium in these vegetables is poorly absorbed)
- Tofu (bean curd) processed with calcium sulfate
- Canned sardines or salmon with bones

Table 1.2 lists other nondairy calcium sources.

Table 1.2 Alternate Sources of Calcium

Food	Amount	Calcium (mg)
Sardines with bones*	3 oz	370
Salmon with bones*	3 oz	170
Shrimp, canned	3 oz	100
Tofu, processed with calcium sulfate**	4 oz; 1/4 cake	145
Molasses, blackstrap	1 T	135
Spinach, cooked	1/2 c	120
Turnip greens, cooked	1/2 c	100
Kale, cooked	1/2 c	90
Bok choy, cooked	1/2 c	80
Target intake		800–1,200 mg/day

*You have to eat the bones to get the calcium! **Read the ingredients on the label. If calcium sulfate is not listed, that brand of tofu is a poor source of calcium.

Note. ''From Composition of Foods'' in *Agricultural Handbook No. 8-4* by the U.S. Department of Agriculture, 1979, Washington, DC: U.S. Government Printing Office.

How Much Calcium

To consume the amount of calcium you need to build and maintain strong bones (800 to 1,500 milligrams per day), you should plan to include a calcium-rich food in each meal. Here are some tips to help you boost your calcium intake to build and maintain strong bones:

- For breakfast, eat cereal with 1 cup low-fat or skim milk (300 milligrams). For crunchy cereal, use yogurt (415 milligrams per cup) in place of milk. For hot cereal, cook the cereal in milk and/or mix in 1/4 cup powdered milk (290 milligrams).

- When planning a quick meal, choose pizza with low-fat mozzarella cheese (150 milligrams per slice), sandwiches with cheese, preferably low-fat (200 milligrams per ounce).
- Make calcium-rich salads by adding grated cheese (200 milligrams per ounce) or low-fat cottage cheese (70 milligrams per 1/2 cup). Use yogurt-based dressings; mix salad seasonings into plain yogurt (415 milligrams per cup).
- Drink low-fat milk with lunch, snacks, or dinner (300 milligrams per cup).
- Add milk instead of cream to coffee (only 15 milligrams per 1 ounce of creamer). Bring powdered milk to the office to replace coffee-whiteners, or drink milk-based hot cocoa (300 milligrams) in place of coffee.
- Snack on fruit yogurt rather than ice cream (315 versus 150 milligrams). Frozen yogurt, ice milk, and puddings are also tasty low-fat calcium treats (150 to 250 milligrams).
- If you're a fish lover, canned salmon or sardines with bones (170 and 370 milligrams respectively per 3 ounces) are easy lunch options; serve with crackers.
- Add tofu (145 milligrams per 1/4 cake) to soups or spaghetti sauce. Read the labels on the tofu containers and be sure to choose the brands processed with calcium sulfate; otherwise the tofu will be calcium-poor.
- Chow down on dark green, leafy vegetables such as spinach, broccoli, and kale (about 200 milligrams per cup).

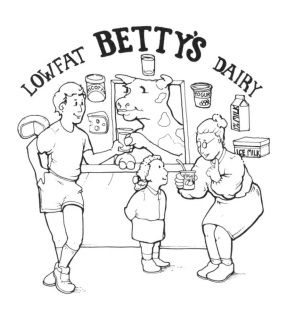

People who have trouble digesting milk because they lack an enzyme (lactase) that digests milk sugar (lactose) need to find alternate calcium sources. Some milk-intolerant athletes can tolerate yogurt, hard cheeses, or even small amounts of milk. Others enjoy Lactaid Milk, a lactose-free brand available at larger supermarkets. I also recommend a nutrition consultation with a registered dietitian to assure appropriate calcium intake.

In most cases, calcium supplements are a poor alternative to calcium-rich dairy products because the calcium from pills is absorbed less effectively than that from milk. Calcium pills also supply far fewer nutrients than power-packed dairy products. For example, milk is one of the best sources of riboflavin, a vitamin that helps convert the food you eat into energy. Active people need more riboflavin than their sedentary counterparts because they generate more energy. If you don't eat dairy products, your riboflavin intake is likely to be poor.

Milk Myths

One high school football player who drank milk by the quart ("I can polish off a half-gallon at one dinner!") was concerned that this much milk would cause calcium deposits. For most healthy people, this is unlikely. When you consume more calcium than your body needs, your body excretes the excess.

Myths abound regarding milk for athletes. For example, one runner thought that milk causes cottonmouth. It doesn't. The dryness he experienced prior to competition was due to nervousness and anxiety, not to milk.

A soccer player had heard that milk is hard to digest and causes stomach cramping. It doesn't, unless you're lactose intolerant. Low-fat milk and dairy products are easy to digest. Little babies can handle milk; so can grown athletes. A *lack* of milk or of adequate calcium may contribute to muscle cramping. One track star was plagued with leg cramps until he started drinking milk again after having avoided it for a year.

There are also milk myths about broken bones. Skiers commonly hobble into my office on crutches, wondering if they would benefit from guzzling gallons of milk. Drinking extra milk does *not* hasten the healing process! Six to 8 weeks and a balanced diet are the two main keys to mending broken bones.

Good Nutrition Game Plan: Fruits and Vegetables

Some best choices: oranges, bananas, melon, broccoli, spinach, green peppers, tomatoes

Suggested minimum intake: 2 large (1 cup) portions* per day (or 4 smaller portions)

Main nutrients: vitamins C and A, potassium, carbohydrates, and fiber

Protective benefits:

- Improve healing
- Reduce risk of cancer, high blood pressure, and constipation
- Aid recovery after exercise

Eat-and-runners often don't get enough fruits and vegetables. Many frustrated business professionals and fitness fans give the following reasons for having unbalanced diets:

- They rarely eat fruit because it's unavailable.
- They don't take the time to cook vegetables or fix salads.

If you have trouble including fruits and vegetables in your daily diet, the following tips will help you balance your intake better and make these foods a top priority in your good nutrition game plan.

Some Top Fruit Choices

If you like fruit but just don't get around to eating it, plan into your breakfast either a banana or orange juice. These are among the most nutritious fruits, so you'll be getting a good start to the day. These fruits are also easily toted.

Citrus Fruits and Juices. Whether whole or fresh, frozen or canned, citrus fruits such as oranges, grapefruit, and tangerines surpass many other fruits or juices in terms of vitamin C and potassium.

If peeling citrus fruit is a bother for you, drinking its juice is an acceptable alternative. The whole fruit has slightly more nutritional value, but given the option of a quick glass of juice or nothing, juice does the job! Just 6 ounces of orange juice provides the daily requirement of vitamin C (60 milligrams) plus all the potassium you might have lost in an hour's workout, plus folic acid, a B vitamin needed for building protein and red blood cells. Orange juice also has fewer calories and more nutrients than many other juices, including cranberry, apple, and grape.

---

*One portion = 1 cup juice; 1 medium-large piece of fruit; medium tossed salad; 1 cup of cooked vegetables

To boost your juice intake, stock up on cans of the frozen juice concentrate, buy juice boxes for lunch or snacks, and look for cans of juice in vending machines. Or better yet, buy whole oranges.

Bananas.   This low-fat, high-fiber, and high-potassium fruit is perfect for busy athletes and nonathletes alike, and even comes prewrapped! Bananas are excellent recovery foods for replacing potassium lost in sweat. To boost your banana intake, include bananas on cereal, pack them into a brown bag for a low-calorie dessert (a medium banana contains only 100 calories), or keep them on hand for a quick and easy energy-boosting snack. My all-time favorite is a banana with peanut butter, stoned-wheat crackers, and a glass of milk—a well-balanced meal that covers all four food groups (fruit, protein, grains, and dairy).

To prevent bananas from overripening, store them in the refrigerator. The skin may turn black from the cold, but the fruit itself will be fine. Another trick is to keep banana chunks in the freezer. These frozen nuggets taste just like banana ice cream with far fewer calories.

Without a doubt, bananas are among the most popular sports snacks. I've even seen a cyclist with two bananas safely taped to his helmet, ready to grab when he needed the energy boost!

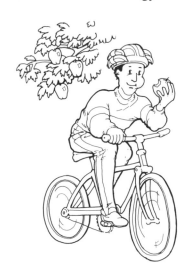

Cantaloupe, Kiwi, and Strawberries.   These nutrient-dense fruits also are good sources of vitamin C and potassium.

Dried Fruits.   Convenient and portable, these are rich in potassium and carbohydrates.

If you aren't eating much fruit, be sure that the fruit you do eat is nutritionally the best. The information in Table 1.3 can help guide your choices.

Some Top Vegetable Choices

In general, vegetables have more nutritional value than fruits; if you aren't a fruit eater or if fruits leave you with an acid stomach, you

Table 1.3   Comparing Fruits

Fruit	Amount	Calories	A (IU)	C (mg)	Potassium (mg)
Apple	1 med	80	75	10	160
Apple juice	1 c	116	0	2	296
Apricots	dried, 10 halves	85	2,535	1	480
Banana	1 med	105	90	10	450
Blueberries	raw, 1/2 c	40	70	10	65
Cantaloupe	1 c pieces	55	5,160	70	495
Cherries	10 sweet	50	145	5	150
Cranberry juice	1 c	147	—	108	61
Dates	5 dried	115	20	—	270
Figs	raw, 1 med	35	70	1	115
Grapefruit	1/2 med, pink	35	320	45	160
Grapefruit juice	1 c	96	—	94	400
Grapes	1 c	60	90	5	175
Honeydew melon	1 c	60	70	40	460
Kiwi	1 med	45	135	75	250
Orange, navel	1 med	65	255	80	250
Orange juice	1 c	111	50	124	496
Peach	1 med	35	465	5	170
Pear	1 med	100	35	5	210
Pineapple	1 c raw	75	35	25	175
Pineapple juice	1 c	139	1	27	334
Prunes	5 dried	100	835	2	310
Raisins	1/3 c	150	4	2	375
Strawberries	1 c raw	45	40	85	245
Watermelon	1 c	50	585	15	185
Target intake			>5,000	>60	>2,000

Note. Nutrient data from *Bowes and Church's Food Values of Portions Commonly Used* (14th ed.) by J. Pennington and H. Church, 1985, Philadelphia: Lippincott. Adapted by permission.

can simply eat more veggies and get the same vitamins and minerals, if not more.

Dark, colorful vegetables usually have more nutritional value than paler ones. For example, the deeper green or deeper yellow a vegetable is, the more vitamin A it contains. If you're struggling to improve your diet, don't stuff yourself with pale lettuces, cucumbers, zucchini, mushrooms, and celery. Instead, feast on colorful broccoli, spinach, green peppers, tomatoes, and carrots, which offer far more nutrients.

Here's the scoop on the top vegetable choices:

Broccoli, Spinach, and Green Peppers. These low-fat, potassium-rich vegetables are loaded with vitamins C and A. One stalk (1/2 cup) of steamed broccoli offers you the RDA for vitamin C, as does half a large green pepper or a spinach salad (4 ounces). I enjoy munching on a green pepper instead of an apple for an afternoon snack; it's got more vitamins C and A, more potassium, and fewer calories. What a nutritional bargain!

Tomatoes and Tomato Sauce. In salads or on pasta or pizza, these are another easy way to boost your veggie intake. Tomato products are good sources of potassium, fiber, and vitamin C (one medium tomato provides half the RDA for vitamin C). Tomato juice and vegetable juice are additional suggestions for fast-laners who lack the time or interest to cook—those speedsters can simply drink their veggies! Tomato products tend to be high in sodium, however, so people with high blood pressure should limit their intake.

Cruciferous Vegetables (Members of the cabbage family). Cabbage, broccoli, cauliflower, brussel sprouts, bok choy, collards, kale, kohlrabi, and mustard greens may be protective against cancer, as may vitamin A–rich choices such as carrots, winter squash, and greens. Surveys suggest that people who consume significant amounts of these vegetables tend to have lower cancer rates. Do your health a favor by focusing on these choices!

Fresh, frozen, and canned vegetables all have similar nutritional value. Of course, fresh from the garden is best but often impossible. Frozen vegetables are a good second choice. Freezing doesn't destroy the nutritional value, overcooking does. Canned vegetables are processed quickly to retain most of their nutrients, which is a plus when you use the vegetable water for soups or stews. To reduce their high sodium level, rinse canned vegetables with plain water.

For more information on vegetables, see Table 1.4.

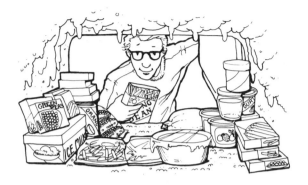

Table 1.4   Comparing Vegetables

Vegetable	Amount	Calories	A (IU)	C (mg)	Potassium (mg)
Asparagus	1 c cooked	30	1,200	40	275
Beans, green	1 c cooked	30	675	15	190
Beets	1/2 c canned	25	4	3	150
Broccoli	2/3 c or 1 lg stalk, cooked	25	2,500	90	270
Brussel sprouts	6–8 med, cooked	35	520	85	275
Cabbage	1 c cooked	35	200	50	230
Cabbage	1 c raw	25	130	50	235
Carrot	1 lg raw	40	11,000	10	340
Cauliflower	1 c cooked	25	70	65	235
Celery	1 stalk, raw	10	120	5	170
Corn	frozen, 1/2 c	90	240	5	195
Cucumber	1/2 med, with peel	10	125	5	80
Kale	1 c cooked	35	9,870	80	290
Lettuce, iceburg	1 wedge	15	330	5	175
Lettuce, romaine	4 lg leaves	20	1,900	20	265
Mushrooms	4 lg raw	30	trace	5	415
Onion	1 med, raw	40	40	10	155
Peas, green	1 c cooked	105	810	30	300
Pepper, green	1 lg shell, raw	20	420	130	215
Potato	med, boiled in skin	75	trace	15	580
Spinach	1 c cooked	40	14,600	50	580
Squash, summer	1 c cooked	30	780	20	280

(Cont.)

Table 1.4   (Continued)

Vegetable	Amount	Calories	A (IU)	C (mg)	Potassium (mg)
Squash, winter	1 c baked	125	8,400	25	920
Tomato	raw, 1 med	35	1,350	35	365
Tomato sauce	1/2 c canned	45	1,200	15	485
Target intake			>5,000	>60	>2,000

Note. Nutrient data from *Bowes and Church's Food Values of Portions Commonly Used* (14th ed.) by J. Pennington and H. Church, 1985, Philadelphia: Lippincott. Adapted by permission.

Good Nutrition Game Plan: Meats and Protein-Rich Alternatives

Some best choices: lean meat, fish, poultry, nuts, beans, legumes

Suggested intake: 4–6 ounces per day* or 2 small servings

Main nutrients: protein, B vitamins, iron and zinc in dark meats

Protective benefits:

- Assure proper muscle development
- Reduce risk of iron-deficiency anemia
- Improve healing

Risks: Fatty meats may contribute to heart disease.

Slabs of beef and huge hamburgers have no place in a sports diet, or in any diet; excess protein isn't stored as bulging muscles or muscle fuel. However, smaller amounts of protein are important for building muscles and repairing tissues. The purpose of this section is to highlight quick and easy protein choices.

The protein rule-of-thumb is to include a total of 4 to 6 ounces of protein-rich food at lunch or dinner or split between these two meals. Four ounces is tiny compared to what most Americans eat—12-ounce steaks, 8-ounce chicken breasts, 7-ounce cans of tuna. Many athletes polish off their required protein by lunchtime and daily eat 2 to 3 times

---

*4 ounces is about the size of a woman's palm or a deck of cards.

what they need. Others, however, miss out on adequate protein when they fuel up only on salads, plain pasta, or stir-fry vegetables; these athletes exclusively load up on carbohydrates *(carbo-load)* and neglect their protein needs.

See chapter 11 for more information on protein needs, vegetarian diets, and muscle-building foods.

Some Top Protein Choices

Although all types of chicken, fish, eggs, and beef are excellent sources of protein, they offer different types of nutrients.

Lean beef. A lean roast beef sandwich made with two thick slices of bread (for carbohydrates) is an excellent choice for iron, which prevents anemia; for zinc, needed for healing; and for B vitamins, which help produce energy. Other nutrients are present as well that are important for the sports diet. In terms of heart health, a lean beef sandwich is preferable to a grilled cheese sandwich, tuna salad, or hamburger because of these nutrients and the lower fat content.

Chicken and Turkey. Poultry generally has less saturated fat than red meats, so it tends to be a more heart-healthful choice. Just be sure to discard the skin (which is all fat). I remove chicken skin before cooking; cooked until crispy, chicken skin can be a big temptation.

Fish. Canned or fresh, fish is not only a great source of protein, but it's also protective against heart disease. The recommended target is three fish meals (canned or fresh) per week, with the best choices being the more oily varieties such as salmon, albacore tuna, swordfish, sardines, and bluefish. However, any fish is better than no fish.

Peanut Butter. Good old peanut butter. What would we do without this "emergency food"? Although peanut butter by the jarful can be a dangerous diet-breaker, a few tablespoons on whole grain bread, crackers, a bran muffin, or banana offers protein, vitamins, and fiber in a satisfying snack or a quick meal. Being a vegetable source of protein, peanut butter has no cholesterol; the old-fashioned brands offer more polyunsaturated (as compared to saturated) oils—two plusses for people concerned about heart health.

Even noncooks can easily incorporate adequate protein into a day's diet. Simply buy lean roast beef, roast chicken, or turkey at the deli counter; open a can of tuna or salmon; or resort to peanut butter, hummus (chick-pea spread—see the recipe in Section IV) or nuts. Other nutritious protein-rich foods include beans, lentils, and legumes. These vegetable proteins can be quick and convenient during your busy week *if* you cook them in quantity on the weekend. Table 1.5 lists some popular protein foods.

Table 1.5   Where's the Protein

You don't have to eat beef to get plenty of protein, but animal products generally provide the highest quality protein. Vegetable sources should be combined with animal proteins to enhance their quality, or combined with other complementary vegetable proteins (see chapter 11).

Food	Serving size	Protein (g)
Animal sources		
Egg	1 lg	6
Milk	1 c	8
Cheddar cheese	1 oz	8
Yogurt	1 c	10
Cottage cheese	1/2 c	14
Codfish, cooked	4 oz	30
Hamburger, cooked	4 oz	30
Chicken, cooked	4 oz	35
Pork, cooked	4 oz	40
Vegetable sources		
Almonds	12–15	3
Peanut butter	1T	4
Chili beans	1/2 c	7
Split peas	1/2 c	7
Lentils	1/2 c	7
Tofu	3 oz	10

Good Nutrition Game Plan: Grains and Starches

Some best choices: cereal, wholesome bread, pasta, rice

Suggested minimum intake: 4 servings* per day

---

*1 serving = a small bowl of cereal, 1 slice of bread, or 1/2 cup of rice or pasta

Main nutrients: carbohydrates, fiber, B vitamins

Protective benefits:

- Fuel muscles
- Protect against needless muscular fatigue
- Fiber reduces problems with constipation
- Low in fat, hence low in calories and good for weight-reduction programs

These foods are the equivalent of gasoline in a car. The trick to a healthy, carbohydrate-rich sports diet is to avoid the fats that generally accompany carbohydrates: butter on bread, cream cheese on a bagel, or oil on fried rice. Low-fat carbohydrate cuisine requires discipline and dedication, especially if you're eating fast foods.

When selecting grains, try to choose the ones that have been only lightly processed, if processed at all. For example, brown rice, whole wheat bread, and stoned-wheat crackers offer more B vitamins, potassium, and fiber than refined white rice, white bread, and white crackers (see Table 1.6). Chapter 7 explains in greater detail the importance of wholesome starches and grains in a sports diet.

Top Carbohydrate Choices

To fuel your muscles with premium nutrition, choose from among the following top carbohydrates.

Table 1.6 Refined Versus Whole Grains

In general, whole grains tend to have more nutritional value than products made from refined flour. This chart compares the nutrients in dark versus light flours.

Bread/2 sl	Fiber (g)	Potassium (mg)	Vitamin B_6 (mg)
Pumpernickel	0.6	280	0.10
Whole wheat	0.6	170	0.10
Light rye	0.2	100	0.04
White, enriched	trace	60	0.02
French	trace	45	0.02
Suggested intake	25–35	>2,000	2.0

Note. Nutrient data from *Bowes and Church's Food Values of Portions Commonly Used* (14th ed.) by J. Pennington and H. Church, 1985, Philadelphia: Lippincott. Adapted by permission.

Bran Cereals.   Bran cereals are rich sources not only of fiber but also of B vitamins and often of iron (if they are enriched with this nutrient). Bran flakes, orange juice, and a banana constitute a real breakfast of champions. See chapter 3 for more information on cereals.

Oat Bran.   Cooked into a tasty hot cereal, oat bran makes a wonderful breakfast that helps lower cholesterol and is protective against heart disease. This microwaveable meal-in-a minute is quick, enjoyable, and good for your health!

Whole Grain and Dark Breads.   When it comes to choosing bread products, remember that whole grain breads tend to have more nutritional value than white breads. At the sandwich shop, request the turkey with tomato on dark rye or whole wheat. At the supermarket, select the hearty brands that have *whole wheat* listed as the first ingredient. Keep them in the freezer so you'll have a supply on hand for sandwiches or toast.

Stoned-Wheat and Whole Grain Crackers.   These low-fat munchies are a perfect high-carbohydrate snack for your sports diet. Be sure to choose wholesome brands with a low fat content, *not* the ones that leave you with greasy fingers! (See Table 1.7).

Table 1.7   Fat in Crackers

Brand or type	% Calories from fat
Ry-Krisp	4
Ak-Mok	18
Zwieback	20
Saltines	21
Uneeda biscuits	21
Oyster crackers	25
Triscuits	32
Wheat Thins	35
Ritz	48
Waverly Wafers	64

Note. Nutrient data from *Bowes and Church's Food Values of Portions Commonly Used* (14th ed.) by J. Pennington and H. Church, 1985, Philadelphia: Lippincott. Adapted by permission.

Muffins and Bagels.   Whole grain muffins (bran, corn, and oatmeal) and bagels (pumpernickel, rye, or whole wheat) are more healthful than white flour–based muffins, donuts, buttered toast, croissants, or danish pastries. A muffin or bagel along with yogurt and orange juice creates a well-balanced meal-on-the-run that's easily available from a convenience store or cafeteria, if not from home.

The Balancing Act

Now that you know which foods are the best choices, the trick is to pull them all together into wholesome meals and snacks. I recommend that you eat selections from at least three of the four food groups at each meal.

Sample Menu	*1*	*2*	*3*
Grain	Bran cereal	Corn muffin	Pizza crust
Dairy	Low-fat milk	Yogurt	Cheese
Fruit/Vegetable	Banana	Orange	Tomato sauce
Protein	(Milk)	Peanut butter	(Cheese)

Pizza (without pepperoni, sausage, or other greasy meats) is an excellent example of a well-balanced meal. Topped with peppers, onions, mushrooms, and other vegetable toppings, it's far from a junk food. It offers calcium (from the low-fat mozzarella), potassium, vitamins A and C (from the tomato sauce and vegetable toppings), fiber (if you can find a pizza made with whole wheat crust), and lots of other nutrients. Given the choice between a fast-food burger or pizza, you'll get more carbohydrates and healthfulness from the pizza. (Caution: If you're on a salt-restricted diet, eat pizza in moderation because it is high in sodium.)

Most people naturally balance and vary their food choices, enjoying a variety of foods and consuming a variety of nutrients. In contrast, Martha, a collegiate athlete, complained that she ate the same foods every day because she hated the school food. She existed solely on corn flakes for breakfast, a turkey sandwich on white bread for lunch, lettuce salad for dinner, and peanut butter on crackers for snacks. I encouraged her to at least eat different brands of cereal topped with different fruits for breakfast, and different types of sandwiches and breads for lunch; to add lots of dark, colorful vegetables to the salad; or, if she preferred to stick to the same old choices, to at least choose from the best foods with the most nutrients:

- Bran cereal, banana, orange juice
- Dark sandwich breads
- Colorful salad veggies

The goal of your good nutrition game plan is simply to choose more of the best and less of the rest!

To form the foundation of eating a well-balanced sports diet, just remember to choose by twos:

- *Two dairy products.* Perhaps low-fat milk on cereal for breakfast, yogurt with lunch (plus two glasses of low-fat milk if you're a growing teen or a postmenopausal or otherwise amenorrheic woman).
- *Two small protein servings.* Perhaps peanut butter on a muffin, and tuna in a sandwich.
- *Two good-sized fruits or vegetables.* Perhaps 8 ounces of orange juice for breakfast and a generous dinner salad.
- *Two thirds of the plate covered with carbohydrates at dinner.* Such as two baked potatoes and a large serving of vegetables, and only one piece of chicken.

CHAPTER 2

Eating Your Way to Health

Nutrition excesses, not deficiencies, are the biggest nutrition problem in America. Excess saturated fat, cholesterol, refined foods, and gooey calories contribute to obesity, heart disease, cancer, hypertension, diabetes, kidney failure, and other diseases of aging.

Fortunately, your daily diet can help protect your health. The same foods you eat to enhance your sports performance also help you maintain your well-being. Everyone wins in the long run with a wholesome, high-carbohydrate, low-fat sports diet!

Eat to Your Heart's Content

Although heart disease is the number one killer in America, sports-active folks often believe they're exempt from "The Low-fat Rules" about heart-healthy eating because they're *athletic*. Being athletic will protect them from heart disease, right? *Wrong*. Even sports-active folks can succumb to heart disease. The sudden death of marathoner Jim Fixx is just one testimonial. Hungry athletes should ration their intake of ice cream, cookies, cheese, and other foods bulging with saturated fat and cholesterol, as should fitness-conscious folks. No one is exempt. Unfortunately, most of us are confused by the constant updates and changes of heart-health information. This leaves us wondering what the real answers are to questions like the following.

Is Beef Good or Bad?

A few years ago, everyone shunned the stuff, believing it to be an artery clogger. Today, health experts tell us that small portions of lean beef aren't so bad, after all, especially for athletes who need beef's iron, zinc, and other important nutrients. Despite popular belief, beef is not exceptionally high in cholesterol; it has a cholesterol value similar to chicken and fish. Beef tends to have more saturated fat than chicken or fish, so that's why it has a bad name among health-watchers. This saturated fat is a bigger culprit than dietary cholesterol. Figure 2.1 defines fat and cholesterol and may help clarify this confusing topic.

Figure 2.1 _____

Definitions: Fat and Cholesterol

Fatty acids are grouped in three families:

saturated
monounsaturated
polyunsaturated

Each fatty acid molecule consists of atoms of carbon, hydrogen, and oxygen arranged in a specific pattern.

When there is a hydrogen at every available spot in the molecule, the fatty acid is *saturated*. It is holding all the hydrogen that is possible; its chemical structure looks like this:

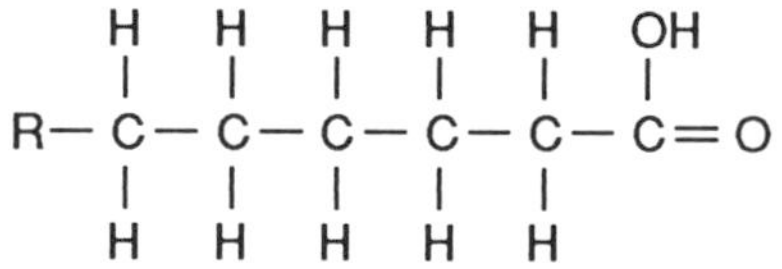

```
      H   H   H   H   H   OH
      |   |   |   |   |   |
  R—  C — C — C — C — C — C=O
      |   |   |   |   |
      H   H   H   H   H
```

When some hydrogen is missing, the molecule is unsaturated. If just one molecule of hydrogen is missing, the fatty acid is *monounsaturated*. Olive oil is a monounsaturated fat.

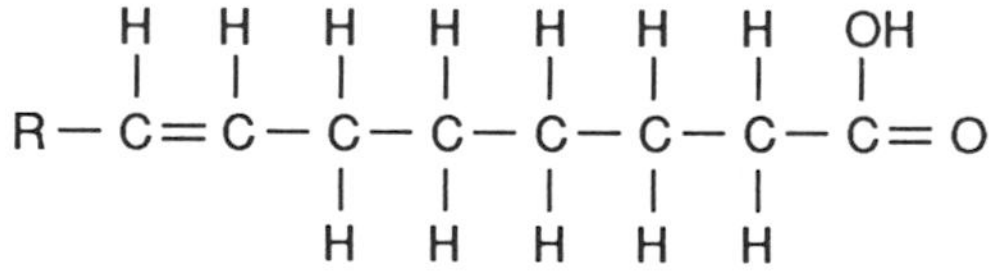

```
      H   H   H   H   H   H   H   OH
      |   |   |   |   |   |   |   |
  R—  C = C — C — C — C — C — C — C=O
          |   |   |   |   |
          H   H   H   H   H
```

If two or more molecules of hydrogen are missing, the molecule is polyunsaturated. Corn oil is a polyunsaturated fat.

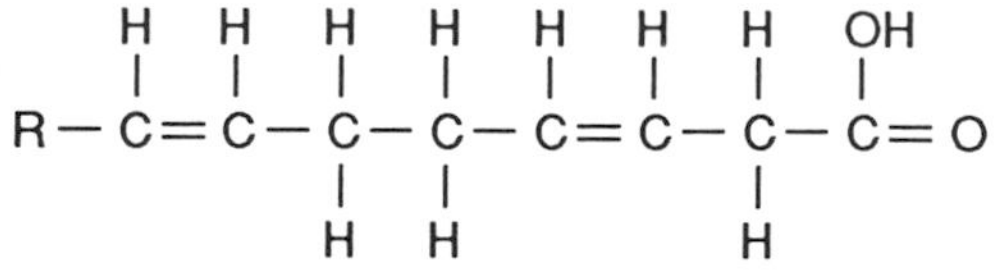

```
      H   H   H   H   H   H   H   OH
      |   |   |   |   |   |   |   |
  R—  C = C — C — C — C = C — C — C=O
          |   |           |
          H   H           H
```

Fatty acids travel in the blood in the form of triglycerides. Three fatty acid chains attach to a molecule of glycerol to form a triglyceride:

Cholesterol is not a member of the fatty acid family. It has a different chemical structure and is not used for energy.

You can fit beef, pork, and lamb into a heart-healthy sports diet if you

- select lean cuts of beef, such as eye of round, rump roast, sirloin tip, flank steak, or bottom round; and
- eat smaller portions; limit yourself to 4 to 6 ounces rather than 16.

Table 2.1 can help guide your choices, and the recipes in Section IV offer low-fat cooking suggestions.

Are Eggs Good or Bad?

Some medical experts tell us that eating eggs is bad because a single egg has 210 milligrams of cholesterol; others report that egg cholesterol

Table 2.1   Fat and Calories in Meat

Saturated fats in animal products can increase your risk for heart disease. To lower your intake of fats and calories, choose leaner cuts of meats.

Meat	% Fat	Calories/4 oz cooked
Beef		
Stew beef	30	210
Round steak	30	215
Flank steak	35	225
Rump roast	40	235
Porterhouse steak	42	255
Rib roast	50	275
Ground beef, regular, broiled	62	325
Lamb		
Roasted, shank half of leg	35	200
Roasted, sirloin half of leg	42	225
Loin chop, broiled	42	235
Pork		
Loin, tenderloin, roasted	25	190
Ham	45	250
Loin, top loin, roasted	50	280
Spareribs, braised	70	450
Veal		
Arm steak, braised	20	215
Sirloin chop, braised	25	220

Note. Reprinted from *Nutrition Action Healthletter*, which is available from the Center for Science in the Public Interest, 1501 16th Street, N.W., Washington, D.C. 20036, for $19.95 for 10 issues, copyright 1988.

may have little effect upon the blood cholesterol level in many people. The American Heart Association currently recommends that we limit our cholesterol intake to 300 milligrams *per day* and a single egg just about hits that limit.

To date, it's unclear whether the cholesterol that you eat affects the amount of cholesterol in your blood because most of the blood's cholesterol is made in the liver. We do know that dietary fats affect the way the body disposes of cholesterol. In particular, saturated fats (such as butter and beef fat) appear to inhibit the body's ability to get rid of the bad form of cholesterol (low-density lipoprotein, or LDL) that clogs arteries. We also know that some people respond more readily than others to a low-cholesterol diet. So, when it comes to eggs, you should limit your intake if you have a high blood cholesterol level and a family history of heart disease; the American Heart Association recommends a limit of three eggs per week *including* those used in cooking. Otherwise, if you have low blood cholesterol and no family history of heart disease, this highly nutritious protein source may be eaten in moderation as part of your balanced nutrition game plan.

Is Oil Good or Bad?

Liquid oils are acceptable fats to include in limited amounts in a heart-healthy diet. In particular, the monounsaturated fats in olive oil and canola (better known by the brand name ''Puritan'') oil seem to be health-protective heroes and perhaps better choices than safflower, corn, sunflower, and other polyunsaturated vegetable oils. Use these oils with salads, pesto, and pasta, and when sautéeing. Just be sure to use only moderate amounts so that most of your calories still come from carbohydrates.

When it comes to selecting vegetable fats, the softer forms—liquid corn oil rather than solid margarine, soft tub margarine rather than stick margarine—have a higher percentage of unsaturated fats and are therefore preferable to fats of animal origin such as butter, bacon grease, and fatty meats. Refer to Table 2.2 for more information about comparing fats.

Table 2.2   Good Fat, Bad Fat

Foods ladened with saturated fat raise your blood cholesterol level. Choose foods with more monounsaturated or polyunsaturated fats instead.

Fat	% Saturated	% Monounsaturated	% Polyunsaturated
Highly saturated vegetable fats			
Coconut oil	90	10	—
Palm oil	50	30	20

(Cont.)

Table 2.2   (Continued)

Fat	% Saturated	% Monounsaturated	% Polyunsaturated
Animal fats			
Butter fat	65	30	5
Beef fat	50	45	5
Chicken fat	30	50	20
Monounsaturated oils			
Olive oil	15	75	10
Canola oil	5	60	35
Peanut oil	20	50	30
Polyunsaturated oils			
Safflower oil	10	15	75
Sunflower oil	10	20	70
Corn oil	15	25	60
Cottonseed oil	25	20	55

Note. From "Composition of Foods" in *Agricultural Handbook No. 8-4* by the U.S. Department of Agriculture, 1979, Washington, DC: U.S. Government Printing Office.

The following tips should help to further dispel confusion regarding the best foods to eat to keep your heart ticking in good health.

Ticker Tip #1: Know Your Number

Know where you stand when it comes to heart disease. By knowing your cholesterol level, you can assess your risk of developing heart disease. Make an appointment with your doctor to get your blood tested for:

Total Cholesterol.   A waxy substance that contributes to hardening of the arteries. Cholesterol accumulates on the walls of the blood vessels throughout the body, especially those in the heart. This buildup limits blood flow to the heart muscle and contributes to heart attacks.

HDL Cholesterol.   *High density lipoprotein* cholesterol, the "good stuff" that carries the bad cholesterol out of the arteries.

LDL Cholesterol.   *Low density lipoprotein* cholesterol, the "bad stuff" that deposits cloggage.

Total Cholesterol to HDL Ratio.   At least 25 percent of your total blood cholesterol should be HDL. Because exercise tends to boost HDL, active people often have a high percentage of this good cholesterol. Their total cholesterol may be higher than that of a sedentary person, but as long as 25 percent of it is HDL these individuals are okay. The higher the HDL percentage, the lower the risk of heart problems.

Desirable Blood Cholesterol Targets

In 1987, the National Institutes of Health recommended that all adults over age 20 have their serum total cholesterol measured at least once every 5 years; this measurement should be made after a 12-hour fast. Following are guidelines for determining who is at risk for heart disease and who needs to carefully monitor their diets. If your total cholesterol is high, you should have it remeasured, looking at both HDL and total cholesterol. Sports-active people often have a high percentage of HDLs.

Desirable levels	<200 mg/dl*
Borderline-high blood cholesterol	200–239 mg/dl
High blood cholesterol	>240 mg/dl

Genetics play a large role in health, so you may have a cholesterol that puts you at a high risk for developing heart disease even if you eat a high-carbohydrate, low-fat diet. One 28-year-old triathlete was shocked to discover his cholesterol was very high. He probably had inherited this trait form his father and grandfather, both of whom had had heart attacks.

Once you know your cholesterol rating, you'll be better able to determine how strict you need to be with your diet. For example, if your level is less than 180 milligrams and if your 97-year-old parents are still alive and thriving, you can perhaps be a bit more lenient than your buddy whose cholesterol is a risky 250 milligrams and whose father suddenly died of a heart attack at age 54.

Ticker Tip #2: Cut the Fat

Eat less fat, particularly saturated animal fat. This means cutting down on, or eliminating from your diet, such things as greasy hamburgers, pepperoni, hot dogs, sausage, full-fat cheeses, and butter. Use small

*mg/dl = the number of milligrams cholesterol per 100 cc of blood.

amounts of olive oil, canola, safflower, or sunflower oils for cooking, rather than butter, lard, or animal fat drippings. Both a sports diet and a heart-healthy diet limit fat to 25 to 30 percent of caloric intake.

The American Heart Association allows 30 percent of daily calories to come from fat:

- 10% from olive or canola oil and other monounsaturated vegetable fats.
- 10% from corn or safflower oil and other polyunsaturated vegetable fats.
- 10% from butter, lard, and animal fats, as well as from coconut and palm oils, two highly saturated vegetable oils that are commonly used in processed foods.

I advise sports-active people to aim for a 25-percent-fat diet. The trade-in of 5 percent of their fat calories allows them to eat more carbohydrates. Hence, if you're an active woman who eats about 2,000 calories per day, 500 of these could come from fat:

$$25\% \text{ fat x } 2,000 \text{ cal } = 500 \text{ cal from fat}$$

If you ration your intake of butter, margarine, mayonnaise, salad dressing, ice cream, cookies, chips, and other obviously high-fat foods, you'll end up with about a 25-percent-fat diet.

Follow these three steps to determine the amount of fat that you can healthfully include in your diet:

1. Estimate how many calories you need per day. See ''Ten Tips for Successful Weight Reductions'' (p. 191) in Chapter 14 for instructions.
2. Multiply your total daily calories by 25 percent (.25) to determine the number of fat calories you can eat.
3. Divide your allotted fat calories by 9 to determine the number of grams of fat you can eat daily. (One gram fat = 9 calories).

For example, if you're entitled to 500 fat calories:

$$500 \text{ fat cal } \div 9 \text{ cal/g } = 55 \text{ g fat}$$

Table 2.3 can help you determine your target fat intake. If you are underweight or very active and need more calories from fat to boost your total caloric intake eat more of the heart-healthy fats, such as olive, canola, or corn oils.

Ticker Tip #3: Read Food Labels

The information on food labels can help you compare the types and amount of fat, and sometimes cholesterol, in specific foods. As you

Table 2.3   Target 25-Percent Fat Intake

For a heart-healthy sports diet, you should target your fat intake to about 25 percent of your total calories.

Calorie needs per day	Grams fat for 25% fat intake
1,200	35
1,500	40
1,800	50
2,000	55
2,400	65
2,600	70

now know, cholesterol is found in the foods we get from animals (dairy products, meats). Cholesterol is *not* present in foods of plant origin (fruits, vegetables, grains, and the like). Thus when you read a label on peanut butter, for example, that seems to shout "Cholesterol-free" at you, well, it's true, but it never had cholesterol in the first place. Some cereal manufacturers do this as well; the labels say their foods are "wholesome" and "natural." Yet, some of these so-called natural grains are processed with coconut and palm oils, which are saturated fats. When you look at a label, note the grams of fat, but also read the ingredients to see what type of fat the food contains. Table 2.4 compares the amount of fat and cholesterol in some common foods.

If you have a very high cholesterol level, your physician may recommend a diet that's 20 percent or even 10 percent fat. This restriction is for people clinically endangered by heart disease, not for healthy folks who already have low cholesterol levels. I often talk to food fanatics with low cholesterol who try to eliminate *all* fats from their diet. They burden themselves with needless restrictions; a low-fat diet need not be a *no*-fat diet.

Ticker Tip #4: Eat More Oats

Oats have a fiber-rich outer bran layer that effectively lowers blood cholesterol. Standard oatmeal is 12 percent fiber, and oat bran is 18 percent fiber. The latest research suggests that 2 ounces of oat bran each day can help people attain low cholesterol levels, especially when eaten within a low-fat diet (Van Horn, 1986).

Oat bran is available in the hot cereal section of many supermarkets and health food stores. It's similar to cream of wheat but has a nutty

Table 2.4   Fats and Cholesterol in Some Common Foods

Food product	Amount	Fat (g)	Cholesterol (mg)
Milk			
skim	1 c	0	5
2% low-fat	1 c	5	20
whole	1 c	8	35
Cheese			
cheddar	1 oz	10	30
swiss	1 oz	10	25
mozzarella			
(part-skim)	1 oz	5	15
ricotta (part-skim)	1 oz	10	35
cottage cheese			
(low-fat, 2%)	1 oz	4	20
Ice Cream			
expensive brands			
(16+% fat)	1/2 c	12-18	40-50
less expensive			
brands (10% fat)	1/2 c	5	30-35
ice milk	1/2 c	3-5	8-10
Lean Meats/Fish			
(cooked)			
pork	4 oz	15	80
beef	4 oz	13	80
lamb	4 oz	11	80
chicken	4 oz	5	70
tuna	4 oz	1	70
shrimp	4 oz	1	220
Cereals			
Quaker 100%			
Natural	1/4 c	5	0
oatmeal, uncooked	1/3 c	2	0
oat bran, uncooked	1/3 c	2	0
Post Grape-Nuts	1/4 c	0	0
Snack and Fast Foods			
potato chips	1 oz	10	0
pretzels	1 oz	1	0
corn/nacho chips	1 oz	7	0
cheese curls	1 oz	10	1

Food product	Amount	Fat (g)	Cholesterol (mg)
McDonald's Egg McMuffin	1 svg	15	230
McDonald's Filet of Fish	1 svg	25	45

Note. Nutrient data from *Bowes and Church's Food Values of Portions Commonly Used* (14th ed.) by J. Pennington and H. Church, 1985, Philadelphia: Lippincott. Adapted by permission.

flavor. Enjoy it as a hot cereal (yummy with chopped almonds and raisins), or bake it into muffins. (See the recipes under "Breads and Breakfasts" in Section IV.)

Although I'd never been a fan of hot cereals, I've now discovered that oat bran is my favorite snack before a morning run. It takes the edge off my appetite and settles comfortably. I cook it effortlessly in the microwave while reading the comics in the morning newspaper, cool it off and make it into a "soup" with low-fat milk, drink it down, read the rest of the paper, and head out the door feeling comfortably fed. Try it. You might like it, too!

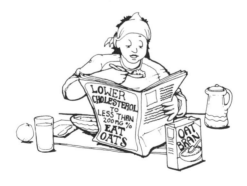

Ticker Tip #5: Eat More Fish

If good health is your wish, get hooked on fish! Current research indicates that fish—particularly the oilier fish that live in cold ocean waters such as salmon, mackerel, albacore tuna, sardines, and herring—guards against not only heart disease but also hypertension, cancer, arthritis, and who knows what else! The omega-3 fatty acids, a special polyunsaturated fat found in fish oil, block many harmful biochemical reactions that can cause blood to clot (predisposing you to heart attack and stroke). Fish oils can *prevent* heart disease from the beginning rather than merely having an effect *after* the disease has set in.

Eating at least two or three fish meals per week may reduce your risk of heart disease. However, not all fish are created equal. Some guard your health better than others. Table 2.5 can help guide your fish choices. Just be sure that your fish is prepared in ways that are healthy for your heart—*not* fried or broiled in butter.

If you're not a fish fan, you may be tempted to take the seemingly easier alternative—fish oil pills. Despite the fancy price tag, these supplements contain only a small amount of omega-3s compared to a fish dinner. For example, you might have to take 10 capsules of one popular brand (at $1 or more) to get the equivalent of a 4-ounce serving of salmon. Health professionals also question whether the supplements are as effective as the fish itself. To date the consensus is to get hooked on fish, not on pills.

Table 2.5   Fish Highest in Omega-3 Fatty Acids

Fish	Omega-3 fatty acids (g/7 oz raw or 5 oz cooked)
Atlantic mackerel	5
King mackerel	4.5
Pacific herring	4
Lake trout	4
Norwegian sardines	3
Bluefin tuna	3
Chinook salmon	3
Albacore tuna	3
Atlantic salmon	3
Sockeye salmon	2.5
Greenland halibut	2

Note. Data from F. Hepburn, J. Exler, and J. Weihrauch. "Provisional Tables on the Context of Omega-3 Fatty Acids and Other Fat Components of Selected Foods." Reprinted from *Journal of the American Dietetic Association,* **86**: 788, 1986.

The Anti-Cancer Crusade

In the United States, cancer follows heart disease as the most frequent cause of death. Diet is a factor in an estimated 35 percent of cancer cases.

Despite the gloomy news that one in four of us will get cancer, the encouraging news is that dietary changes can prevent perhaps one third of cancer deaths. Your sports diet wins again! The low-fat, high-fiber, top-performance sports diet can also be a cancer-protective diet that may reduce your risk of developing this dreaded disease.

Protective Nutrients

One key to the role of diet in preventing cancer may lie in an antioxidative capacity—that is, in a nutrient's ability to deactivate harmful chemicals in the body known as *free radicals*. Free radicals are formed daily through normal body processes. Environmental pollutants—such as cigarette smoke, automobile exhaust, radiation, and herbicides—also generate free radical precursors. These unstable compounds can attack, infiltrate, and injure vital cell structures. Fortunately, our bodies have natural control systems that deactivate and minimize free radical reactions within the cells. These natural control systems involve many vitamins and minerals, including these:

- *Beta-carotene*, a form of vitamin A found in plants and converted into vitamin A in the body, helps prevent the formation of free radicals.
- *Vitamin C* guards against harmful reactions within the cells.
- *Vitamin E and selenium* protect the cell walls from free radical damage. Selenium also enhances the immune system's response with increased resistance to cancer growth.

To boost your intake of these anti-cancer nutrients, you should focus your diet on foods such as these:

- Dark green and colorful vegetables rich in vitamin A, such as broccoli, spinach, carrots, and leafy greens
- Members of the cabbage family (cruciferous vegetables), such as cauliflower, broccoli, kohlrabi, bok choy, and brussel sprouts
- Vitamin C–rich foods, such as grapefruit, oranges, melon, strawberries, broccoli, and spinach
- Whole grain foods rich in vitamin E, including whole wheat bread, wheat germ, nuts, and peanut butter
- Selenium-rich foods, such as tuna, nuts, lean meats, and seafood

Refer to Table 2.6 for more information about these protective nutrients.

Table 2.6   The Fantastic Four

High intakes of several nutrients (selenium and vitamins A, C, and E) can possibly help reduce the incidence of cancer. But they're best available in food, not supplements. This chart shows where to get foods rich in these nutrients.

Selenium (RDA not established)	Vitamin A (RDA = 5,000 IU)	Vitamin C (RDA = 60 mg)	Vitamin E (RDA = 7–13 mg)
An adequate amount of selenium is between 50 and 200 micrograms, and the best food sources are seafood, meats, and grains. The selenium content of foods varies with regional differences in the selenium content of soil and water. Supplements are not recommended due to danger of toxicity (with long-term supplementations over 200 micrograms).*	The best food sources are green and yellow vegetables. The conservative recommendation for cancer prevention is 12,500 IU.* Two active forms include retinol and beta-carotene. Retinol may have toxic effects with long-term supplementation greater than 25,000 IU. Beta-carotene, in excess, affects skin color by turning it yellow, a common occurence if you eat too many carrots.	The best sources are fruits and vegetables. There is only a neglible risk of toxicity in ascorbic acid, the chemical name for vitamin C. The conservative recommendation for cancer prevention is 1,000 mg.*	The best sources are vegetable oils (and foods made with them such as salad dressing and baked goods), nuts seeds, and whole grains. The RDA refers to Alphatocopherol, the most active form of vitamin E. There is a negligible possibility of toxicity. Doses higher than 800 mg can cause toxic symptoms including nausea, diarrhea, and intestinal cramps. The conservative recommendation for cancer prevention is 200 to 800 mg.*

Common sources

Selenium	mcg	Vitamin A	IU	Vitamin C	mg	Vitamin E	mg
Tuna, 1/2 can (3.5 oz)	115	Carrots, 1 lg raw	11,000	Orange juice, 1 c	120	Sunflower seeds, 1/4 c	13
Codfish, 4 oz	50	Carrots, 1/2 c cooked	7,600	Grapefruit juice, 1 c	100	Safflower oil, 1 T	8
Chicken thigh, 3-1/2 oz	40	Spinach, 1/2 c cooked	7,200	Broccoli, 2/3 cooked	90	Sunflower oil, 1 T	7
Noodles, 1 c cooked	40	Winter squash, 1/2 c	4,300	Orange, med	80	Almonds, 1 oz	4
Spaghetti, 2 oz dry	35	Cantaloupe, half	3,300	Brussel sprouts, 6–8	70	Peanuts, 1 oz	2
Molasses, 1 T	35	Broccoli, 1 lg stalk	2,500	Green pepper, 1/2	65	Spinach, 1/2 c cooked	2
Cashews, 1 oz	20	Apricots, 2 dried	1,600	Strawberries, 10 lg	60	Olive oil, 1 T	1
Skim milk, 1 c	12	Tomato sauce, 1/2 c	1,100	Cauliflower, 1 c cooked	60	Tomato, 1 lg	1

*Information from Watson & Leonard (1986). Table reprinted by permission of Runner's World (The Runner) magazine, March 1987.

Research suggests that a high intake of selenium and vitamins A, C, and E can potentially reduce the incidence of some types of cancer. Most health professionals emphasize the importance of obtaining these nutrients from food, not from supplements. "The nutrients should not be viewed as cure-alls that work alone," according to Watson and Leonard (1986, p. 505). "Adequate intake should be the result of increased dietary consumption rather than supplements because of yet unidentified components in food that may prove beneficial and protective."

Cancer and Fat

Eating a low-fat diet may be a second dietary key to reducing cancer risk. Population studies suggest that people who eat high-carbohydrate, low-fat diets have a lower incidence of cancer. The National Research Council recommends that we eat less than 30 percent of our total calories as fat, eat more fruits and vegetables rich in vitamins C and A (refer to Tables 1.4 and 1.5 for the nutrients in fruits and vegetables), as well as eat more whole grains. This sounds like a high-carbohydrate sports diet to me!

In addition to thinking about food's relationship to cancer, you should also think about your lifestyle. You can guard your good health not only by eating wisely but also by exercising and having a healthy mental outlook. As Don Ardell (1986) says in his book *High Level Wellness: An Alternative to Doctors, Drugs, and Disease,*

There are many factors that contribute to optimal health. Nutrition is *one* very important factor. But relaxation, peace of mind, positive outlook on life, contented spirit, absence of envy, love of mankind and faith are all-powerful, health promoting factors without which optimal health cannot be achieved. (p. 135)

This holistic approach to cancer prevention includes nourishing yourself with pleasant, high-carbohydrate, low-fat meals; enjoying exercise as a part of your daily routine; and taking time to smell the daisies.

Shake It or Leave It: Salt and High Blood Pressure

High blood pressure, or hypertension, affects approximately 25 to 30 percent of all Americans. Your physician can determine if you fall within this category by measuring your blood pressure: The normal range is 120 over 80, and pressures that exceed 165 over 95 are considered high.

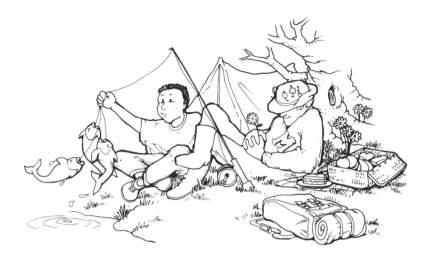

Many health-conscious people believe that salt causes high blood pressure and that reducing salt intake prevents it. Recent studies, however, suggest this is not always the case (Weinberger, 1988; Dairy Council Digest, 1984; Tufts University Diet & Nutrition Letter, 1988).

Of those Americans diagnosed as having high blood pressure, there is a known cause for only 10 percent. The remaining 90 percent have no exact cause, but may exhibit risk factors that can predispose them to the condition, including obesity, smoking, high stress, poor kidney function, and poor diet. Most health-conscious exercisers are not obese, do not smoke, and eat a better-than-average diet, thus eliminating several risk factors. However, additional predisposing factors—such as your genetic makeup, age, and race—cannot be changed.

It is true that for some people too much sodium, combined with any or all of the other risk factors, may raise blood pressure to an unhealthy level. But before you put yourself on a very-low-salt diet, you need to know (1) your own blood pressure, and (2) your family's history of high blood pressure.

If you suspect that you may be at risk for hypertension, you should see your doctor to get an accurate diagnosis. Then, if you are found to have high blood pressure, talk to your doctor and a registered dietitian about a sodium-restricted diet.

Because sports-active people lose salt when they perspire heavily, a low-salt diet may be a needless restriction for those with normal-to-low blood pressure readings and no family history of hypertension. Yet if you are in this group, you needn't worry about harmful effects from cutting back on salt; your body will adjust by conserving more sodium and secreting less. Less salt *may* benefit your long-term health, but the answer is not clear-cut.

What Is Salt?

Salt is a compound made of 40 percent sodium and 60 percent chloride. The sodium in salt is the main concern when it comes to high blood pressure. This mineral helps maintain proper fluid balance in and around your body's cells; thus, you do need some sodium—1,000 to 3,000 milligrams per day. Most Americans, however, consume three to seven times this amount!

Tips for Hypertensives

If you and/or your relatives have high blood pressure, your best bet is to restrict your salt intake to about 2,000 to 3,000 milligrams sodium per day, or about 1 milligram per calorie (one teaspoon of salt has 2,300 milligrams of sodium). You can do this by following these guidelines:

Shaking the Salt Habit

Foods to Avoid:

Table salt—Sprinkled on food and used in cooking. Train your tastebuds to appreciate the flavor of unsalted foods.

Obviously salty foods such as salted crackers, potato chips, pretzels, popcorn, salted nuts, olives, pickles and sauerkraut.

Smoked and cured meats and fish such as ham, bacon, sausage, corned beef, hot dogs, bologna, salami, pepperoni, lox, and pickled herring. Processed cheeses are also higher in sodium than natural brands.

Seasonings and condiments such as catsup, mustard, relish, Worcestershire sauce, steak sauce, soy sauce, MSG, and garlic salt.

Commercially prepared foods—Canned or frozen meals, dried mixes, bouillon cubes (unless labeled "low-sodium" or "sodium-free").

Baking soda, seltzers, and antacids. Some laxatives may be high in sodium.

Cooking Tips:

Omit or reduce salt from cooking and baking. You can leave it out without affecting the outcome. Substitute wines and vinegars for salt.

Experiment with different herbs and spices. When you try a new
seasoning, cautiously add a small amount rather than over-
season. Some tried-and-true combinations include:

Beef—Dry mustard, pepper, sage, marjoram; red wine or sherry

Chicken—parsley, thyme, sage, tarragon, curry; white wine or
vermouth

Fish—Bay leaf, cayenne pepper, dill, curry, onions, garlic

Eggs—Oregano, curry, chives, pepper, tomatoes, pinch of sugar

Foods to Select	Approximate Sodium Content	Comments
Milk, yogurt (preferably low-fat)	125 mg/c	
Cheese (preferably low-fat)	200 mg/oz	Moderate amounts; 1–2 oz/day
Meat, poultry, fish	20 mg/oz	
Eggs	60 mg/egg	
Fruit, juice	5 mg/serving	
Vegetables	10 mg/serving	Fresh and frozen. If canned, rinse well.
Breads	150 mg/sl	
Cereal (cold)	250 mg/serving	
Margarine, butter	50 mg/pat	
Baked goods	250 mg/serving	Once a day, if at all.

Rather than focusing just on sodium to alleviate high blood pressure, you should perhaps pay more attention to potassium, a protective mineral. Eating a potassium-rich diet seems to guard against
hypertension and may control blood pressure more effectively than
a low-sodium diet does. Potassium helps make arteries stronger and
better able to withstand the blood vessel damage that can occur with
aging.

A wholesome, carbohydrate-rich sports diet generally includes
potassium-rich foods. See Table 2.7 for the potassium content of some
familiar foods.

Calcium is another mineral that helps protect against high blood
pressure. For a list of calcium-rich foods, refer to Tables 1.1 and 1.2.

Table 2.7   Potassium Content of Some Common Foods

Potassium is found in most wholesome foods—fruits, vegetables, whole grain breads and cereals, lentils, beans, nuts, and protein foods. Refined or highly processed foods, sweets, and oil foods (salad dressing, butter, etc.) are poor sources of potassium. You can increase your potassium intake by eating the following kinds of foods:

- *Whole wheat, oatmeal,* and *dark breads* instead of white bread and flour products.
- More *salads* and *raw vegetables,* or *steamed veggies* cooked in only a small amount of water because the potassium leaches into the water. Steaming removes only 3 to 6 percent of the potassium, as compared to 10 to 15 percent with boiling.
- *Potatoes* more often than rice, noodles, or pasta.
- *Natural fruit juices* instead of fruit-flavored beverages or soft drinks.

The suggested daily intake for potassium is 2,600 milligrams for the average person and 6,000 for the athlete not acclimatized to the heat. The typical American diet contains 4,000 to 7,000 milligrams of potassium. One pound of sweat loss may contain 85 to 105 milligrams.

Foods	Potassium (mg)
Fruits	
Banana, sm 6″	370
Prunes, 5 dried	350
Orange, med	300
Cantaloupe 1/4 melon	250
Apple, med	165
Raisins, 2 T	150
Pear, med	65
Vegetables	
Tomato sauce, 1/2 c canned	590
Mushrooms, 4 raw	415
Tomato, med raw	365
Carrot, 1 raw	340
Spinach, 1/2 c cooked	290
Broccoli, 1 stalk cooked	270
Lettuce, 1 wedge iceburg	265
Pepper, green, 1	215
Beans, green, 1 c cooked	190
Peas, 1/2 c cooked	125
Protein Foods	
Hamburger, lean 4 oz	550
Chicken, white meat 4 oz	470
dark meat, 4 oz	365

Foods	Potassium (mg)
Fish, haddock, 4 oz	405
Tuna, 1/2 c	280
Peanut butter, 2 T	250
Egg, 1 med	60
Cereals, Grains, and Starches	
Potato, baked	750
Flour, whole wheat, 1 c	445
Beans, kidney, 1/2 c canned	350
Wheat Chex, 1 c	160
Bran flakes, 1 c	135
Spaghetti, 2 oz raw, 1 c cooked	115
Flour, white, 1 c	105
Rice, brown, 1/4 c raw	105
Oatmeal, 1/3 c dry	95
Bread, whole wheat, 1 sl	65
Rice, white, 1/4 c raw	45
Bread, white, 1 sl	25
Cornflakes, 1 c	25
Dairy Products	
Yogurt, 1 c fortified low-fat	530
Milk, 1 c whole or low-fat	380
Cheese, cottage, 1 c low-fat	220
Ice Cream, 1 c	220
Cheese, cheddar, 1 oz	25
Beverages	
Orange juice, 1 c	420
Apple juice, 1 c	240
Beer, 12 oz	90
Cranberry juice, 1 c	25
Gatorade, 1 c	25
Coke, 12 oz	5

Note. Nutrient data from *Bowes and Church's Food Values of Portions Commonly Used* (14th ed.) by J. Pennington and H. Church, 1985, Philadelphia: Lippincott. Adapted by permission.

Salt for Athletes

Even sweaty athletes who prefer the natural taste of unsalted food can get adequate sodium from the sodium that occurs naturally in foods. For the most part, your body adapts to the heat by conserving salt and sweating proportionately more water. If you are unacclimatized to the heat, as on that first warm spring day when you overex-ercise to clear out the winter cobwebs, you'll notice that your sweat is far saltier than at the end of the summer when you've adapted to the heat. If you really need salt, you will crave it. Many ultra-marathoners and long-distance cyclists munch on salted crackers, chips, pretzels, and other salty snacks to satisfy their salt cravings.

For more information on salt and potassium for athletes, see chapter 9.

Fiber: Jumping on the Bran Wagon!

Fiber is the part of plant cells that humans can't digest. Having heard claims that fiber promotes regular bowel movements, lowers blood cholesterol, and protects against colon cancer, sports-active Americans are seeking out high-fiber, carbohydrate-rich foods—the fruits, vegetables, beans, legumes, and whole grains that easily fit into a sports diet.

Certain types of fiber have specific health benefits. For example, the *insoluble fiber* in wheat bran relieves constipation and may help prevent cancer. Wheat bran absorbs water, increases fecal bulk, and makes the stool easier to pass. By tripling stool volume, fiber dilutes the concentration of bile acids, substances that digest fat and are suspected cancer instigators. Some researchers believe that bile acids irritate the intestinal lining leaving it open to attack from carcinogens. A high-fiber, low-fat diet may reduce by 30 percent your risk of developing colon cancer, and with a fiber-rich diet that promotes regular bowel movements you'll feel more comfortable during training and competitions. The information in Table 2.8 can help you choose the foods richest in fiber.

The *soluble fiber* in beans, legumes, and oat bran lowers blood cholesterol. In one study (Van Horn, 1986) about 2 ounces of oat bran were added to a low-fat, low-cholesterol diet, and subjects' serum cholesterol dropped 5 percent. Keeping in mind that a 1-percent drop in serum cholesterol reduces by 2 percent your risk of heart disease, the subjects lowered their risk by 10 percent. You can try to do the same by eating more oatmeal breads, oatmeal cookies, and oat bran muffins as well as hot oat bran cereal. Eating more beans and legumes will also help, and these are also excellent sources of carbohydrates and protein. Corn bran, barley, and rice are other rich sources of soluble fiber that are becoming more readily available.

Despite popular belief, fiber does not hasten the time it takes for food to pass through your digestive system. It may increase fecal

Table 2.8   Fiber in Foods

Fiber is lost through food processing such as milling whole wheat into white flour, peeling skins, puréeing vegetables, and juicing fruits. To reach the target intake of 25 to 35 grams of fiber per day, you should try to eat foods that have not been processed. You should also try to eat a *variety* of fiber-rich foods because different types of fibers have different positive health effects.

Product	Fiber (g)
Cereals, 1 oz	
All Bran	10
40% Bran Flakes	5
Fruit and Fibre	5
Shredded Wheat	3
Granola	trace
Legumes, 1/2 cup	
Kidney beans	6
Split peas	5
Lima beans	5
Vegetables, 1/2 c	
Peas	4
Brussel sprouts	4
Corn	4
Potato	4
Mushrooms	1
Lettuce	trace
Grains	
Brown rice, cooked, 1/2 c	2.5
Whole wheat bread, 1 sl	1.5
Spaghetti, cooked, 1/2 c	1.0
White bread, 1 sl	0.5
White rice, 1/2 c	0.1
Fruits	
Prunes, 3 dried	4
Apple with skin, med	2.5
Banana, med	2
Peach, med	1.5
Raisins, 2 T	1.3
Grapes, 12	0.5

Note. Nutrition data from *Plant Fiber in Foods* by J. Anderson, Lexington, KY: HCF Nutrition Research Foundation, Inc. Adapted by permission of James W. Anderson, MD.

weight and the number of trips to the bathroom, but generally not transit time. Transit time varies for each person but normally averages between 2 and 4 days. This varies according to stress, exercise, and diet. Your best bet, as an active person, is to determine the right combination of fiber-rich foods that promotes regular bowel movements for your body. You may need to restrict your fiber intake if exercise itself becomes a powerful bowel stimulant.

Building Strong Bones for Life: Calcium and Osteoporosis

Osteoporosis, or thinning of the bones with aging, results in hunched backs and brittle bones that break easily. It is a serious health problem primarily among older, postmenopausal women, but also among younger female athletes who have stopped having regular menstrual periods. Both groups lack adequate estrogen, a hormone that contributes to menstruation and helps to maintain bone density.

You can reduce your risk of developing osteoporosis with a lifelong calcium-rich diet and regular exercise program. Unfortunately, too many women skimp on one or both of these areas. I once counseled a very thin 24-year-old amenorrheic runner who had the bones of a 60-year-old. She rarely drank milk (believing it to be merely a fattening fluid), ate a very restrictive low-calorie, low-protein diet, and was always trying to be thinner despite her obvious leanness. Little did she know that this low-protein, low-calorie diet was contributing to the amenorrhea, and that she was putting herself at risk of developing stress fractures—an early sign of poor bone health and premature osteoporosis. She thought that running would keep her bones strong because she'd heard that weight-bearing exercise helps to maintain bone density. Exercise does help, but calcium and estrogen are essential.

Her doctor advised her to regain her menstrual period to protect her bones. Because lack of menstruation can be linked to inadequate nutrition, I taught her how to eat a nonfattening diet that included calcium-rich low-fat milk and yogurt, more protein, and adequate calories. Within 2 months she regained her menstrual period and started promoting her lifelong health.

In chapter one, I talked about how to include in your daily diet the calcium necessary for lifelong fitness. Unfortunately, the typical 25-to 40-year-old woman consumes only 600 milligrams of calcium daily, less than the current RDA of 800 milligrams and the suggested safe intake for women of 1,000-1,500 milligrams. This may be one reason why an estimated 25 percent of women over 65 years are afflicted by osteoporosis (of whom 12 percent may die from medical complications). These women might have reduced their risk by consuming more calcium-rich foods throughout their lifetimes.

Elderly men also may lose enough bone calcium to suffer from osteoporosis. Regardless of gender, those who want to live a long and healthy life should make sure that they promote their future well-being by eating a calcium-rich diet today!

Coffee: Grounds for Controversy

Some folks never touch coffee: "It makes me hyper and jittery." Others thrive on the stuff: "I'm useless without my morning brew."

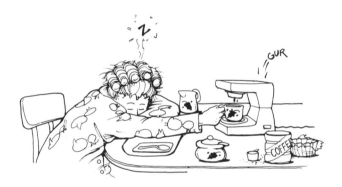

Coffee, like tea and cola, contains the stimulant *caffeine*. Many research studies have tried to link coffee or caffeine to increased risks of cancer, high blood pressure, heart disease, and fibrocystic breast disease. The only confirmed correlation, to date, is that coffee drinkers who smoke cigarettes *do* have a significantly higher incidence of heart disease.

There are others who should abstain from caffeine:

- *Ulcer patients* and others prone to stomach distress. Caffeine stimulates gastric secretions and may cause "coffee stomach."
- *Pregnant and nursing women.* Caffeine readily crosses the placenta and stimulates the unborn infant. Caffeine also crosses into breast milk and can make babies agitated and poor sleepers.
- *Anemic athletes.* Substances in coffee and tea can interfere with the absorption of iron. A cup of coffee consumed with a hamburger can reduce by about 40 percent absorption of the hamburger's iron. If you suffer from anemia and routinely drink coffee or tea with meals or up to 1 hour after a meal, you might be

cheating yourself nutritionally. However, drinking caffeine beverages an hour before eating seems to have no negative effect on iron absorption.

If you are healthy, a moderate amount of coffee (1 or 2 cups per day) is unlikely to harm your health. If you're feeling guilty about your traditional morning mugful, relax and enjoy it. The biggest health worries about coffee have to do with the habits surrounding that beverage:

1. *Adding cream or coffee whiteners containing coconut oil.* These add saturated fat that contributes to heart disease. At least switch to milk for whitening your coffee.
2. *Drinking coffee **instead** of eating a wholesome breakfast.* A large coffee with two creamers and two sugars contains 70 nutritionally empty calories. Multiply that by three mugs, and you could have had a nutritious bowl of cereal for the same calorie price!
3. *Drinking coffee to keep you alert.* A good night's sleep would be a better investment.

These stresses are more likely to harm your health than the caffeine itself.

However, if you're drinking so much coffee that you're nervous, jittery, irritable, and sleep poorly, then you should slowly cut back. Don't try to abstain cold turkey because you're likely to suffer a withdrawal headache. Try reducing your caffeine intake by drinking more of the following caffeine-free alternatives:

- Decaffeinated coffee
- Decaffeinated tea
- Herbal teas
- Hot water with a lemon wedge
- Postum, Pero, and other cereal-based coffee alternatives
- Broth, boullion (low sodium or regular)
- Alba, Ovaltine, and other hot milk-based drinks
- Mulled cider
- Hot cranberry juice

Without a doubt, the best caffeine-free alternative to a coffee break is an exercise break. A quick walk and some fresh air may be far more effective than another cup of brew. The next time you start to feel drowsy, try stimulating yourself with exercise rather than caffeine. For more information about caffeine and performance, see chapter 8.

CHAPTER 3

Breakfast: Your Fast Break to a Better Sports Diet

When it comes to eating a high-energy sports diet, I firmly believe that breakfast is *the* most important meal of the day. You've heard that from your mother, teachers, health professionals, coaches, and the media, ad infinitum—and now you'll hear it from me!

Of all the nutritional mistakes you might make, skipping breakfast is the biggest. Jan, an aerobics teacher, learned this the hard way: She fainted from low blood sugar during one of her morning classes. After teaching a 7:30 class, she felt tired and hungry. With no snack to boost her energy, she plunged into the 9:00 session and soon found herself on the floor surrounded by her frightened students. She had blacked out because she had no fuel for exercise.

Jan's story is a dramatic example of how skipping breakfast can sabotage your sports performance. A high-energy breakfast sets the stage for a high-energy day. Nevertheless, many sports-active people come up with familiar excuses for skipping the morning meal:

- "I don't have time."
- "I'm not hungry in the morning."
- "I don't like breakfast foods."
- "I'm on a diet."
- "If I eat breakfast, I feel hungrier all day."

Excuses, excuses. If you skip breakfast, you're likely to concentrate less effectively in the late morning, work or study less efficiently, feel irritable and short-tempered, or fall short of energy for your afternoon workout. For every flimsy excuse to skip breakfast, there's an even better reason to eat it. Keep reading!

You DO Have Time for Breakfast!

"I just don't have time to eat breakfast. I get up at 5:30, go to the swimming pool, train for an hour, then dash to school by 7:45." Obviously, Brian's morning schedule didn't allow him to relax and enjoy a leisurely meal. However, he still needed the energy to tackle his high school classes.

I reminded him that breakfast doesn't have to be a sit-down, cooked meal. It can simply be a substantial snack after swim practice while riding to school. I advised Brian to plan and prepare a breakfast-to-go the night before. If he could make time to swim, he certainly could make time to eat right for swimming.

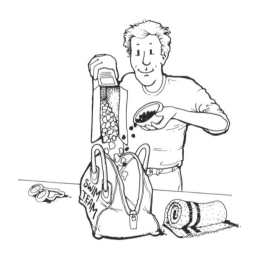

Brian discovered that his "duffle bag breakfast" was indeed worth the effort. Two peanut butter and banana sandwiches and two juice boxes satisfied his ravenous appetite and improved his ability to concentrate at school. No longer did he sit in class counting the minutes until lunch and listening to his stomach grumble. Rather, he was able to concentrate on his classwork and even improve his grades.

Jane, a runner and nurse, had the same excuse of "no time for breakfast." She'd rise at 6:00 and be at the hospital by 6:45; she didn't want to eat breakfast at that early hour. However, by 10:00 she'd be ravenous and devouring doughnuts—grease bombs that she didn't particularly like but that she ate anyway because they were in the nurses' station begging to be eaten!

I recommended that Jane eat some nutritious food between 8:00 and 9:00 to prevent the overwhelming hunger that contributed to her overeating and subsequent weight gain. Jane made the effort to do one of the following every day:

- Bring to work banana bread with peanut butter
- Buy a corn muffin, milk, and juice at the coffee shop
- Take an early break and eat a hot breakfast at the cafeteria
- Keep emergency food in her locker—crackers, nuts, and dried fruits

She soon became a breakfast advocate, feeling so much better when well-fueled rather than half-starved.

If you lack creative quick-fix breakfast ideas, these suggestions can help you make a fast break into becoming a regular breakfast eater:

- *Yogurt*—Keep your refrigerator well stocked; add cereal for crunch.
- *Banana*—Extra large, wash down with a large glass of milk.
- *Blender drink*—Whip together juice, fruit, and dried milk or yogurt.
- *Raisins and peanuts*—Prepacked in small plastic bags.
- *Bran muffin*—Add peanut butter for a heartier treat.
- *Bagel*—With low-fat cream cheese and a can of V-8.
- *Graham crackers*—A favorite with low-fat milk.
- *Pita bread*—Stuff with lite cheese, cottage cheese, peanut butter, or other handy fillings.

No Morning Appetite?

If you're not hungry for breakfast, perhaps you ate too many calories the night before. I often counsel athletes who routinely devour a whole bag of chips while watching TV or raid the cookie jar at 2 a.m. These snacks can certainly curb a morning appetite, contribute to weight gain, and even result in dietary deficiencies (if too many munchies replace wholesome meals).

Mark, a 35-year-old runner and computer programmer, wasn't hungry for breakfast for another reason: His morning workout killed his appetite. However, he did get hungry by 10:00 when his appetite came to life again. He'd try to hold off until lunchtime but raided the candy machine 3 out of 5 workdays. I recommended that Mark take a bagel, yogurt, and/or banana to work. These portable foods are much more nutritious than candy, especially for breakfast!

For morning excercisers like Mark, a wholesome breakfast, such as cereal, fruit, whole grain toast, pancakes, and/or muffins, promptly replaces the depleted glycogen stores and invests in the next training session. Exercised muscles are hungriest for carbohydrates within the first 2 hours after a workout. For more information on recovery foods, see chapter 9.

This recovery breakfast is particularly important if you do two workouts per day. Unfortunately, too many athletes who do double workouts say they're not hungry for breakfast after the first workout. They also skimp at lunchtime, afraid that a substantial meal might interfere with the afternoon session. They end up dragging themselves through a poor workout.

In this situation, I recommend having brunch or a substantial snack around 10:00 or 11:00. The food will be adequately digested in time to fuel the muscles that afternoon. You'll discover that you have more energy for the second workout.

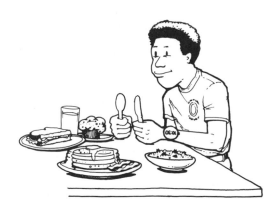

Breakfast for Dieters

Skipping breakfast to save calories is an unsuccessful approach to weight loss. Research indicates that breakfast skippers struggle more with weight than breakfast eaters. You burn breakfast calories more easily than the same amount eaten at night.

In one study with subjects who needed about 2,000 calories per day to maintain their weights, the subjects all lost weight when they ate those 2,000 calories at one morning meal (Halberg, 1983). When they moved these calories to an identical meal in the evening, four of the six gained weight; the other two lost less than they had when they ate breakfast only. The weight-loss difference averaged about 2-1/2 pounds. If you're tempted to save calories by skimping on breakfast, remember that you don't gain weight eating this meal. You do gain weight if you skip breakfast, get too hungry, and then overindulge at night.

Time and again I advise dieters to eat during the day and diet at night. Time and again they look at me with fear in their eyes. As Pat, a weight-conscious dancer, explained: "If I eat breakfast, I get hungrier and seem to eat more the whole day." Her breakfast was a mere slice of 50-calorie diet toast, enough to "prime the pump" and get the digestive juices flowing, but not enough to satisfy her appetite. When she ate a substantial 500-calorie breakfast, she felt fine and didn't blow it late in the afternoon. The following chart provides sample 500-calorie breakfast suggestions, appropriate for an intake of 1,500 calories per day.

Sample 500-Calorie Breakfasts

Breakfast at home	Approximate calories
1 c orange juice	100
2 oz cereal	220
1 c low-fat milk	100
1 small banana	80
Total	500
Breakfast on the run	
Bran muffin, med-lg	300
Vanilla yogurt	200
Total	500
Non-traditional breakfast	
2 slices pizza	
(leftover from dinner)	500
Total	500

Pam, a 28-year-old mother, tennis lover, and self-described life-long dieter, insisted that eating breakfast triggered her to overeat the whole day. I requested she experiment for just 3 days to determine if a substantial 500-calorie breakfast really did make her hungrier and fatter.

Pam quickly discovered that she no longer craved french fries at lunch and that she snacked less in the afternoon, played better tennis after work, and was able to enjoy a relaxed dinner rather than ravenously wolfing down the most quickly available foods the minute she walked in the door. She felt less hungry and snacked less throughout the night. By trading in the evening's 600 to 800 snack calories for 500 breakfast calories, she discovered that breakfast, for her, could become the most important meal of the day!

If you are watching your weight and overeat at breakfast, don't continue to overeat the rest of the day. Compensate by eating less at lunch and dinner. You won't be hungry! Just listen to your body rather than to your mind, which often says that you might as well keep eating because this is your last chance before *The Diet* starts again.

Nontraditional Breakfasts

If you skip breakfast because you don't like breakfast foods, simply eat something else. Who said you have to eat cereal or eggs? Any food you eat at other times of the day can be eaten at breakfast. I happen to love leftover pizza or Chinese food for a morning change of pace!

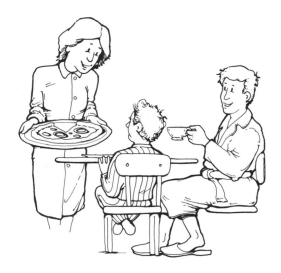

Your goal is to eat about one third of your daily calories in the morning, so you might want to eat a dinner or lunch at breakfast. Try leftovers, a baked potato, a peanut butter and honey sandwich, a cottage cheese "sundae" with sliced fruit and sunflower seeds, tomato soup with crackers, or even special holiday foods; save some of those high-calorie treats that may be left over from a special event and enjoy them for breakfast. You're better off eating them during the day and burning off their calories than holding off until evening, when you may succumb to overconsumption in a moment of weakness!

The #1 Breakfast for Champions

My sports-active clients commonly ask what I recommend for breakfast. My #1 choice is cereals because they are all these positive things:

- *Quick and easy*. Athletes of all ages and cooking abilities can easily enjoy a bowl in a minute with no cooking or messy cleanup.
- *Convenient*. By simply stocking the cupboard, school locker, or desk drawer, breakfast will be ready for the morning rush.
- *Carbohydrate-rich*. Your muscles need carbohydrates for energy. Cereal, a banana, and juice constitute a superior carbohydrate-rich meal.
- *Fiber-rich*. When you select bran cereals, you reduce your risk of becoming constipated, an inconvenience that can certainly interfere with optimal sports performance, and you also consume a health-protective, anti-cancer food.
- *Iron-rich*. By selecting fortified or enriched brands, you can easily boost your iron intake and reduce your risk of becoming anemic. Drink orange juice or another source of vitamin C with the cereal to enhance the iron absorption from the cereal.
- *Calcium-rich*, when eaten with milk or yogurt (preferably low-fat). Women, in particular, benefit form this calcium-booster that helps maintain strong bones and protects against osteoporosis.
- *Low in fat and cholesterol*. Cereals are a heart-healthier choice than the standard breakfast alternative, bacon and eggs.
- *Versatile*. Rather than getting bored by always eating the same brand, try mixing cereals to concoct endless flavors. I typically have 10 to 18 varieties in my cupboard. My friends laugh when they discover this impressive stockpile! I further vary the flavors by adding different mix-ins, such as banana, raisins, applesauce, cinnamon, maple syrup, or vanilla extract.

The Scoop on Cereals

Cereal, in general, is a breakfast for champions. However, some brands offer far more nutritional value than others. Here are five tips to help you make wise choices.

Choose Iron-Enriched Cereals.   An iron-rich diet is particularly important for active people because iron is the part of the red blood cell that carries oxygen from your lungs to your muscles. If you are anemic (have iron-poor blood), you'll feel tired and fatigue easily during exercise. Iron-rich breakfast cereal is a handy way to boost your iron intake.

Most breakfast cereals have iron added to them, as you can determine by looking for the words "fortified" or "enriched" on the label, or by checking the nutrient-information panel to make sure a particular brand supplies at least 25 percent of the U.S. RDA. Table 3.1 pro-

Table 3.1   Nutritional Value of Some Commonly Eaten Cereals

Cereal	Amount per oz	Calories	% Cals from sugar	% Cals from fat	Fiber (g)	Iron (% US RDA)
All-Bran	1/3 c	70	29	13	10	25
40% Bran Flakes	2/3 c	90	22	0	5	100
Cap'n Crunch	3/4 c	120	40	15	—	25
Cheerios	1 1/4 c	110	4	16	2	45
Corn Bran	2/3 c	120	20	7	5	45
Corn Flakes	1 c	100	7	0	1	10
Cracklin' Bran	1/2 c	110	25	33	5	10
Crispy Wheats, Raisins	3/4 c	110	36	8	—	25
Frosted Flakes	3/4 c	110	40	0	—	10
Fruit & Fibre	1/2 c	90	31	10	5	25
Fruitful Bran	2/3 c	110	40	0	4	100
Grape-Nuts	1/4 c	110	11*	0	2	15
Honey Nut Cheerios	3/4 c	110	36	8	—	25
Life	2/3 c	120	20	15	—	45
Nutri-Grain Wheat	2/3 c	100	8*	0	3	4
Product 19	1 c	100	12	0	1	100
Puffed Wheat	1+ c	50	0	0	trace	trace
Quaker 100% Natural	1/4 c	140	17	39	—	4
Raisin Bran (Kellogg's)	3/4 c	120	33**	8	5	100
Rice Krispies	1 c	110	11	0	—	10
Shredded Wheat	2/3 c	110	0*	8	3	6
Special K	1 c	110	11	0	—	25
Total	1 c	110	11	8	2	100
Wheat Chex	2/3 c	100	8	0	2	25
Wheaties	1 c	110	11	8	2	25

* Naturally occurring sugar   **Includes raisins   Compiled from information provided on the cereal boxes, 1988.

vides information that can help you select brands enriched with iron to supplement the small amount naturally occurring in grains.

Because the iron in cereal is often poorly absorbed, you will enhance *iron bioavailability*—your body's ability to absorb iron—by drinking some orange juice or eating fruit rich in vitamin C along with the cereal (try oranges, grapefruit, cantaloupe, and strawberries).

If you prefer all-natural cereals with no additives, remember that "no additives" means that there is no added iron, as is the case with Nutrigrain, Grape-Nuts, shredded wheat, puffed rice, and other all-natural brands. If you like, you can mix all-natural cereals with iron-enriched varieties (for example, Grape-Nuts with Cheerios, granola with Raisin Bran, shredded wheat with Wheat Chex), or you can choose iron-rich foods at other meals or take an iron supplement (for more information on iron, see chapter 12).

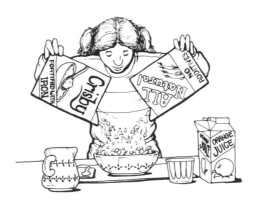

Choose High-Fiber Bran Cereals.   Fiber is beneficial for people with constipation. Recent research suggests that fiber also has protective qualities that may reduce your risk of colon cancer and heart disease.

Bran cereals can provide far more fiber than most fruits and vegetables. High-fiber brands include All-Bran, 40% Bran Flakes, Fruit 'n Fibre, Corn Bran, Raisin Bran, Oat Bran, and any of the multitude of cereals with *bran* in the name. You can boost the fiber content of any cereal by simply sprinkling on raw bran.

Choose Wholesome Cereals.   Some kids' cereals are 45 percent sugar, more dessert than breakfast. Although sugar does fuel the muscles and is not the poison it's reputed to be, sugary cereals tend to pamper your sweet tooth rather than promote your health.

By reading the nutrient information on the cereal box, you can determine a cereal's sugar content:

- Look for *grams of sucrose.*
- One gram of sucrose contains 4 calories.
- Multiply grams by 4 to get total sugar calories.

Wheat Chex and Nutrigrain have only 8 calories (2 grams) of added sugar per ounce, compared to Frosted Flakes, which has 40 calories (10 grams). To put this in perspective, one level teaspoon of sugar is 4 grams (16 calories).

Peter, a 32-year-old cyclist and stockbroker, avoided all cereals with sugar listed among the ingredients, even the lightly sweetened brands such as Life, Wheaties, or Fruit 'n Fibre. He restricted himself to sugar-free Puffed Wheat, Grape-Nuts, and shredded wheat, cheating himself of both iron and fiber. He failed to recognize that sugar is a carbohydrate that fuels, rather than poisons, the muscles.

The 10 to 15 sugar calories in one ounce of cereal are relatively insignificant compared to the sugar Peter ate in ice cream, cookies, and M&Ms. The overall healthfulness of the cereal breakfast far outweighed those few nutritionally empty sugar calories. Given this perspective, he decided to loosen up his sugar rules to include more variety, especially iron-rich brands, with health-protective fiber.

Choose Low-Fat Cereals. Rather than fretting about a cereal's sugar content, you should be focusing on its fat calories. Fat is the bigger health threat because its linked with heart disease and cancer, as well as weight gain. Some brands, particularly granola-types, contain a significant amount of fat, usually coconut or palm oil, added to enhance the texture and provide crunch. These fats are highly saturated and can contribute to heart disease.

Some health food stores also sell granola made with less-saturated oils. Cereals highest in fat include Quaker 100% Natural (39 percent fat), Sun Country Granola (35 percent fat, but no coconut oil), and Cracklin' Oat Bran (30 percent fat). A low-fat alternative to granola is muesli, a whole grain cereal that's popular in Europe and is available here under brand names such as Alpen, Familia, or Mueslix.

Choose Low-Salt Varieties. This is especially important if you are on a very strict low-sodium diet for high blood pressure. Even the higher sodium cereals can fit into a moderate sodium intake (3,000 to 4,000 milligrams). Almost any cereal is a lower sodium alternative to breakfast pastries, muffins, or bacon.

Sodium in Cereals

Although some cereals are relatively higher in sodium than others, their sodium content is still within reasonable limits of a low-sodium (2,000 milligram) diet. By eating 2 ounces of the high-sodium brands plus 1 cup of low-fat milk (125 milligrams), you'll consume 700 milligrams of sodium—less than one third of the day's allottment for a person with high blood pressure.

Cereal	Sodium (mg/oz)
Corn Flakes (Kellogg's)	290
Cheerios (General Mills)	290
Wheaties (General Mills)	270
Raisin Bran (Kellogg's)	230
Nutri-Grain Wheat (Kellogg's)	170
All-Bran (Kellogg's)	260
Raisin Bran (Post)	180
Grape-Nuts (Post)	170
100% Natural (Quaker)	20
Muesli (Familia)	2
Muesli (Alpen)	2
Shredded Wheat (Nabisco)	trace
Puffed Rice (Quaker)	trace

Note. Data from the nutrition labels on the cereal boxes (1988).

Cereal Alternatives

Cereal may be one breakfast of champions, but it's not the only one. For you non–cereal eaters, rest assured that other breakfasts can fuel you for a high-energy day. See the recipes in Section IV for some wholesome, high-carbohydrate breakfast breads you might want to enjoy with a glass of low-fat milk and some fruit or juice.

Whatever your choice, always remember that *any* breakfast is better than *no* breakfast, and a wholesome, *high-carbohydrate* breakfast is best for your sports diet. Amen.

CHAPTER 4

Snacks and Snack Attacks

Many people live on snacks. Jean, a swimmer, office manager, and part-time graduate student, typically

- swims between 6:30 and 7:30 in the morning,
- grabs something for breakfast on her way to work,
- has a hectic day at the office with little time to stop and eat,
- energizes on emergency food filed in her desk drawer,
- works out at the health club before dinner,
- picks up dinner on the way to night school or munches on whatever's around the house, and
- eats a "real meal" once a week—Sunday dinner with her family.

The rest of the time, she snacks, grazes, and munches.

Jean's eating patterns are common to many Americans. A 1985 Gallup poll indicated that for many people snacks contribute 20 to 50 percent of daily calories. Snacking and grazing are replacing the traditional three, well-balanced meals. So it's important that healthy choices become the backbone of a high-snack diet.

Is Snacking Bad?

Despite popular belief, snacking can be good for you *if* you make wise choices. Obviously if you snack on glazed donuts, Twinkies, M&Ms, chips, and cola, you'll fuel yourself with sweets and grease that lack the nutrients you need for optimal performance. The same way that a car needs gasoline *and* spark plugs to function, your body needs calories *and* the vitamins, minerals, and proteins found in wholesome foods.

Wise snack choices include many nutritious and conveniently available items. Jean did a super job of balancing her nutrient intake, despite her hectic schedule and lack of traditional meals. Her choices often included:

- **Breakfast**: Corn muffin and yogurt
- **Lunch**: Pizza with green peppers
- **Emergency munchies**: Peanut butter, wheat crackers, V-8 juice
- **Take-out dinner**: Chinese stir-fried chicken with vegetables and boiled rice
- **Hot dinner at home**: Tomato soup and toasted cheese sandwich
- **Cold dinner at home**: Cereal with a tall glass of orange juice (the breakfast she never ate that morning).

The following list provides additional ideas for snacks and grazing.

Some Healthful Snacks— At Home and On the Road

Dry cereal: Mix your favorite cereal with raisins, dried fruits, cinnamon—or nothing! Some good "finger cereals" include Chex, shredded wheat, Cheerios, puffed wheat, and Life.

Popcorn: Eat plain or sprinkled with spices such as chili powder, garlic powder, onion powder, or soy sauce. If you like, spray with Pam or special low-calorie butter-flavored sprays for the spices to stick. (See the recipes in Section IV.)

Muffins: Preferably homemade so that they will have less fat. If store-bought, choose wholesome bran or corn muffins rather than ones made with white flour (See the recipes in Section IV).

Fruits: Apples, oranges, bananas—any fresh fruit. When traveling, pack along dried fruit for concentrated carbohydrates.

Frozen fruit bars: A pleasant treat that you can slowly savor in good health.

Crackers: Stoned-wheat, Ak Mok, sesame, bran, Ry-Krisp, and others with a low fat content (see Table 1.7).

Bagels, pretzels: Preferably whole grain varieties for more vitamins and minerals along with the carbohydrates.

Baked potatoes: Microwave ovens make these a handy snack. Tasty either warm or cold.

Nuts, seeds: Peanuts, pistachios, almonds, sunflower seeds, pumpkin seeds, and other nuts and seeds are excellent for protein, B vitamins, and vitamin E.

Snack Attacks

I always plan for an afternoon snack to boost my energy. This helps me concentrate better by maintaining my blood sugar level; it also takes the edge off my appetite and fuels me for my afterwork bike commute. I pack the snack along with lunch and take the time to eat it.

Not snacking can be a bad practice. You can get too hungry and later overeat. I've learned that if I don't snack on four crackers at the office, I can very easily eat 20 crackers the minute I get home from work!

Snacks prevent not only hunger sensations but also sweets cravings. Snack attacks, not snacks per se, are the nutritional concern. Many athletes think they're hopelessly, and helplessly, addicted to sugary snacks. Based on my experiences, I believe they are *not* addicted and that they can change their behavior. In fact, I've helped many clients resolve their problematic sweets cravings easily and painlessly. The solution is simple: Eat before you get too hungry. When you are ravenous, you tend to crave sweets and overeat.

If you frequently experience uncontrollable snack attacks, examine the following case studies and solutions to learn how to tame the cookie monster within you.

SNACK ATTACK #1. The Predinner Cookie Binge

"I have the worst sweet tooth. I manage to fight sweets cravings all day. But then when I get home, I inevitably attack the chocolate chip cookies. I feel as though I'm powerless and have no control over sweets. I hope that you can put me on the straight and narrow."

David, 47-year-old marathon runner, accountant, and father

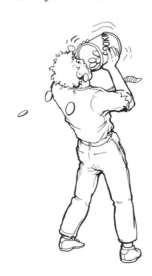

David's story is typical of many of my clients. He came to me feeling guilty about his lack of control over sweets. He required about 3,000 calories per day, but ate zero calories at breakfast and got only 200 from a yogurt at lunch. No wonder he was uncontrollably ravenous by the time he got home—he had accumulated a 2,800 calorie deficit! Nature took control by encouraging him to eat more than enough so that he'd get adequate energy into his system.

I suggested that David eat his 2,500 cookie calories in the form of wholesome meals during the day. He started eating 800 calories for breakfast (cereal, milk, banana, juice, and muffin) and 1,000 calories for lunch or snacks (two yogurts, two large bananas, two juices). Within one day he discovered that he wasn't a cookie monster after all. He could come home, feel untempted by cookies, and have the energy, patience, and desire to cook a wholesome meal rather than grab the handiest foods in sight. He also fueled his muscles better with wholesome carbohydrates rather than buttery cookies. Table 4.1 lists the calories and fat in some popular cookies.

Table 4.1   Calories and Fat in Cookies

You may think you have a sweet tooth when it comes to cookies, but the way most cookies crumble, you may be feeding your "fat tooth." If you succumb to being a cookie monster, at least choose the lower-fat brands!

Name	Brand	Calories/cookie	% Cals from fat
Pecan Sandies	Keebler	80	55
Lido	Pepperidge Farm	90	55
Milano	Pepperidge Farm	65	50
Lorna Doones	Nabisco	35	45
Chips Ahoy!	Nabisco	50	45
Oreos	Nabisco	50	50
Sugar Wafers	Nabisco	20	40
Nilla Wafers	Nabisco	20	30
Animal Crackers	Nabisco	10	30
Social Tea	Nabisco	20	30
Ginger Snaps	Nabisco	30	25
Fig Newtons	Nabisco	50	20
Honey Grahams	Nabisco	30	15

Note: Data from February, 1988, *Tufts University Diet and Nutrition Newsletter*, **5**, p. 12. Adapted by permission.

SNACK ATTACK #2. Premenstrual Sweets Cravings

"Premenstrual chocolate cravings do me in. I can devour a big bag of M&Ms with no problem! I can easily tell 'the time of the month' by my eating habits."

Clarissa, 19-year-old collegiate gymnast

Clarissa, like many women, recognized that her eating patterns changed with the stages of her menstrual cycle. The week before her period she had overwhelming sweets cravings; the week afterwards she tended to crave more protein-type foods, or else had very little hunger. Researchers have verified these eating patterns and report that a complex interplay of hormonal changes seems to influence women's food choices. High levels of estrogen may be linked with the premenstrual carbohydrate cravings.

Women also may crave carbohydrates because they are hungrier. During the week before menstruation, a woman's metabolic rate may increase by 200 to 500 calories daily. That's the equivalent of another meal! However Clarissa, like most women, felt bloated and fat (due to premenstrual water-weight gain) and inflicted upon herself a reducing diet. The result? A double deprivation:

1. The physiological need for extra calories
2. The calorie-deficient reducing diet

No wonder she experienced overwhelming hunger and sweets cravings.

I told Clarissa not to diet but instead, when she felt hungry in the week before her period, to give herself permission to eat 200 to 500 additional wholesome calories each day. She started adding a slice of toast and jam to her standard breakfast, a hot cocoa at lunch, and an afternoon snack of some raisins. She successfully curbed the nagging hunger that had previously plagued her and she was less irritable. She also lost interest in M&Ms and was thrilled to survive a menstrual cycle without gaining weight from chocolate gluttony. See Table 4.2 to discover how quickly those chocolate calories can add up!

SNACK ATTACK #3. Chocolate Addictions

"My diet is atrocious. I simply love chocolate. I'm perfectly content to have brownies for lunch with a Snickers for dessert!"

Paula, 17-year-old high school soccer player

Some folks simply love sweets. They need an excuse to indulge in sugary goo. They eat sweets daily, 3 times if not more: chocolate-frosted donuts for breakfast, brownies for lunch, candy bar for snack, sweet and sour pork for dinner, ice cream sundae for dessert, plus whatever cookies might cross their paths. Needless to say, this high

Table 4.2   Calories and Carbohydrates in Candy

If you're destined to eat candy, limit it to a fun food for a dessert after exercising rather than having it as a "first food" for a meal replacement.

Brand	Amount	Calories	% Cals from carbohydrates
Jelly beans	10 pieces	65	100
Gum drops	28 pieces	100	100
Peppermint Pattie	1 oz	125	80
Milky Way	2.1 oz	260	65
M&Ms	1.6 oz	220	55
Snickers	2 oz	270	50
Mars Bar	1.7 oz	230	50
M&M Peanuts	1.7 oz	240	45
Cadbury Milk Chocolate	1 oz	150	45
Hershey Krackel	1.2 oz	180	45
Reese's Peanut Butter Cup	2 pieces	185	40

Note. Nutrient data from *Bowes and Church's Food Values of Portions Commonly Used* (14th ed.) by J. Pennington and H. Church, 1985, Philadelphia: Lippincott. Adapted by permission.

consumption of sweets results in a poor diet because these sweets lack vitamins and minerals.

Being a healthy, sports-active teen, Paula's diet had space to balance in some sweets without jeopardizing health. For people eating more than 1,700 calories per day, I generally allow for 10 percent of the calories to come from empty calories, if desired. Because she required 2,800+ calories per day, Paula could certainly balance in a 150-calorie cola.

Sweets *abusers* are more at risk for nutritional problems than those who enjoy an occasional treat. There's a big difference between eating a little chocolate as a fun food for dessert after a nourishing meal and eating boxes of chocolates to replace that meal.

Chocoholics often skip breakfast because they're not hungry in the morning. That's because they ate the *whole* bag of chocolate chip cookies the night before. They would nourish themselves better by eating one or two cookies for a bedtime snack and then being hungry for a wholesome breakfast the next morning.

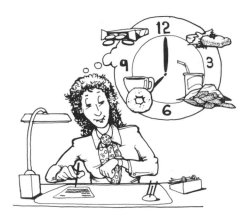

In Paula's case, the chocolate problem stemmed from no time for breakfast, dislike of school lunch, and easy access to the vending machine. I encouraged her to eat breakfast on her way to school, which helped her consume less chocolate during the day.

SNACK ATTACK #4. The "Sugar Fix" Before Exercise

"I'm trying very hard to lose weight, and I am careful about what I eat during the day. However, by the time I leave work for my 5:00 aerobics class, I'm drained and searching for a quick energy boost. I choose something light, like a Coke or apple juice, but I still get that sugar low during class. Any suggestions?"

Priscilla, 37-year-old sales clerk, dieter, and aerobics dancer

When it comes to needing quick energy for the afternoon workout, be cautioned that eating a high-sugar food 30 to 60 minutes before you exercise might have a negative effect. The sugar in soft drinks and even in fruit juices offers a short-term energy boost that later may hinder performance by contributing to *hypoglycemia* (low blood sugar) during exercise.

A concentrated dose of sugar (either natural sugar in fruit juice or refined sugar in soft drinks and jelly beans) rapidly boosts your blood sugar but simultaneously triggers the pancreas to secrete an abnormally large amount of insulin. Insulin transports excess sugar out of the blood and into the muscles. Exercise, like insulin, similarly enhances this transport. Thus, your blood sugar can drop to an abnormally low level once you start to exercise. Some athletes seem more susceptible than others to this rebound hypoglycemia.

Such was the case with Priscilla. Within 10 to 15 minutes after beginning the aerobics class, she felt light-headed, shaky, uncoordinated, and unmotivated to continue. Some days she even had to stop

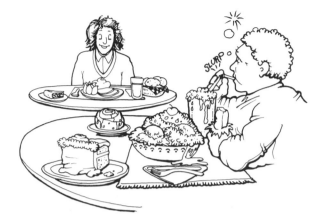

for a rest. The rapid drop in blood sugar—the sugar high followed by the sugar low—interfered with her ability to exercise.

This negative reaction to sweets eaten before exercising was documented by exercise physiologist Dr. David Costill in 1977. He reported that runners who drank 300 calories of sugar (the equivalent of two cans of soft drink) 45 minutes before a hard workout experienced a 19-percent performance decline compared to the same exercise test without the preexercise sugar snack (Costill, 1977).

More recently, a similar experiment resulted in no hypoglycemic effect (Hargreaves, 1987). This study, along with those of other researchers, suggests that some athletes may be more sensitive to sugar than others. My experiences agree with this theory. Among my clients, some describe themselves as being very sugar sensitive; others have never experienced a hypoglycemic reaction after eating sweets.

The safest solution for an energy boost is to maintain a high energy level throughout the day by eating adequate calories at breakfast and lunch. If you haven't done that and you are hungry and craving sweets, eat your sweets within 10 minutes of exercise to avoid the insulin effect. Be aware, however, that you may experience an upset stomach!

In Priscilla's case of a late-afternoon droop, I suggested that she trade her quick-fix calories for more lunch calories. That did the trick. She had an extra half sandwich at lunch (150 calories) instead of an afternoon can of cola (150 calories) and enjoyed her higher energy level.

SNACK ATTACK #5. "The Sugar Fix" During Exercise

"On weekends, I take long bike rides. After about 1-1/2 hours, I start to grind away and feel tired and hungry. My quick fix is a candy bar."

Charlie, a 54-year-old magazine publisher

Although eating sugar before exercise may put you at risk of experiencing a hypoglycemic reaction, eating sugar *during* exercise is unlikely to have a negative effect (other than possible intestinal distress, if the sugar should settle poorly). Exercise supresses insulin secretion; this minimizes the risk of rebound hypoglycemia. Sugar taken during exercise enters your bloodstream and actually prevents you from feeling tired, a key symptom of hypoglycemia. For cyclists, cross-country skiers, ultra-runners and others who exercise for more than 90 minutes, frequent snacks can enhance your stamina.

Some athletes like the natural sugars from fruits and juices, some hit the candy bars, and others prefer sports drinks. Experiment to determine what works best for you. Also experiment to learn how much is appropriate. Research suggests that the body can use about 240 calories of sugar per hour of intense exercise (Coggan & Coyle, 1987). Some athletes can tolerate that much, others can't.

Also keep in mind that too much sugar or food taken at once can slow down the rate at which fluids can leave the stomach to become available to your body for replacing sweat losses. Be more conservative with your sugar fixes in hot weather than during the cold winter, when the risk of becoming dehydrated is lower. Chapter 8 offers more information on nutrition for exercise.

Snacks, Sweets, and Snack Attacks: The Bottom Line

Here are the key points you should remember about snacking:

1. Snacks can be an important part of your training diet; they help prevent you from becoming overwhelmingly hungry. Remember: When you get too hungry, you may not care about what you eat, and you may blow your good intentions on grease and goo.

2. A sugary treat can fit into a well-balanced diet. There's nothing wrong with a cookie eaten for dessert after lunch. The nutrition problem arises when you have cookies *for* lunch.

3. If you find yourself craving sweets, determine whether you've eaten adequate calories to support your activities. The chances are that you've let yourself get too hungry. Sweets cravings are simply a sign that you're physiologically ravenous. To prevent this craving, eat more calories at breakfast and lunch (and snack in the afternoon if you eat a late dinner), so that you curb the cookie monster that tends to arise in the late afternoon and evening.

4. Although a sugar fix before exercising may result in hypoglycemia and fatigue, sugar taken during exercise (<240 sugar calories/hour) can actually enhance performance if you're working for longer than 90 minutes.

CHAPTER 5

How To Build
a Better Sports Salad

Salads are popular among health-conscious, sports-active people. In summertime, salads are a welcome meal because you can toss almost any food into a bowl and create dinner in a hurry without slaving over a hot stove. Or you can stop by your favorite salad bar and enjoy a heaping-good lunch or dinner. For Ginger, a traveling salesperson and squash player, salads offer one hope for a healthful diet. ''I try very hard to eat at restaurants that have a salad bar brimming with all sorts of fresh veggies and fruits. This helps me compensate for my hit-or-miss meals on the road.''

Karin, a collegiate gymnast, also likes salads. ''I hate the cafeteria food at my school, so I live on salads. I only wish their salads contained more than wilted lettuce and squished tomatoes.''

Salad Surprises

Although deemed to be a nutritious blessing, some salads are not what they're thought to be. For example, a bowl of pale vegetables (such as iceburg lettuce, celery, cucumbers, onions) smothered in dressing offers little more than oil and crunch; a McDonald's garden salad (90 calories) becomes decadent when blanketed with the 400 calories in a packet of Thousand Island dressing. You consume more protein, carbohydrates, and less fat with a plain quarter-pound hamburger:

- **McDonald's salad with dressing**: 490 calories—11 percent from carbohydrate, 83 percent from fat.

- **McDonald's Quarterpounder** (with no cheese): 425 calories—30 percent from carbohydrate, 25 percent from fat.

Typically, Americans think of salads as being healthy and low in calories. Dietary analyses suggest that a typical salad-bar meal can easily contain 1,000 calories—43 percent from fat and 45 percent from carbohydrates. In a healthy sports salad, 60 to 70 percent of the calories are from carbohydrates, and at most 25 percent are from fat. This helps explain why many salad-eating exercisers complain of chronic fatigue. They're eating too few carbohydrates to fuel their muscles and support their sports program.

A New Leaf on Life

To create a high-energy sports salad that's the mainstay of your meal, use high-carbohydrate foods and limit the fats. These five tips can help you get the most in your salad bowl:

1. To boost the salad's carbohydrate content, add

    - carbohydrate-dense veggies such as corn, corn relish, peas, beets, and carrots;
    - beans and legumes such as chick-peas, kidney beans, and three-bean salad;
    - cooked rice, pasta, or potato chunks;
    - oranges, apples, raisins, bananas, and berries;
    - toasted croutons (limit your intake of those buttered croutons); and
    - thick slices of whole grain bread, and a glass of low-fat milk, for accompaniments.

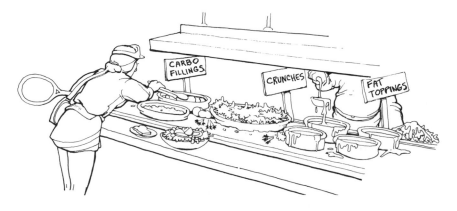

2.   Choose dark, colorful veggies. Salads radiant with red tomatoes, green peppers, orange carrots, and dark lettuces nutritionally
surpass those made with paler lettuces, cucumbers, onions, celery,
and radishes. For example, a salad made with spinach has 6 times
the vitamin C of one made with iceberg lettuce. Dark romaine has
twice the vitamin C (see Table 5.1).
   In general, colorful veggies have more nutrients than pallid ones
(see Table 1.4). Exceptions include beets and corn; although colorful,they have fewer vitamins. Nevertheless, (pickled) beets and corn
(relish) are good choices to boost the carbohydrate value of salads.
Cauliflower, although colorless, is a good source of vitamin C (75 milligrams per cup, raw).

Sports Salad Versus Wimpy Salad

Wimpy salads are primarily pale lettuce drowned in salad dressing—
little more than ''greasy crunch.'' Sports salad are filled with colorful, vitamin-rich vegetables, carbohydrates, protein-rich beans, and
a ''lite'' dressing.

Wimpy Salad	Calories from Carbohydrates	Total Calories
3 c iceberg lettuce	15	20
1/2 lg tomato	20	25
5 T blue cheese dressing	—	400

Total: 445 calories, 10% from carbohydrates, and 90% from fat

Sports Salad	Calories from Carbohydrates	Total Calories
3 c romaine lettuce	15	20
1/2 lg tomato	20	25
1/2 green pepper	8	10
1/2 c broccoli	15	20
1/2 carrot	17	20
1/3 c chick-peas	80	115
1/2 c three-bean salad	65	75
1/3 c toasted croutons	70	80
2 T ''lite'' blue cheese dressing	10	70

Total: 435 calories, 70% from carbohydrates, and 10% from fat

Table 5.1   Salad Fixings

Salad ingredient	Vitamin C (mg) (RDA = 60)	Vitamin A (IU) (RDA = 5,000)	Magnesium (mg) (RDA = 400)
Broccoli, 5″ stalk	110	2,500	24
Green pepper, 1/2 lg	65	210	20
Spinach, 2 c	50	8,100	90
Tomato, med	35	1,380	20
Romaine lettuce, 2 c	20	1,900	20
Iceburg lettuce, 2 c	5	330	10
Cucumber, 1/2 med	5	125	5
Celery, 1 stalk	5	120	10

3.   Salads can easily heighten your intake of potassium, a mineral that not only is lost in sweat but also protects against high blood pressure (see chapter 2). You should try to get at least 2,000 milligrams of potassium each day—an easy task for salad lovers. These are some of the veggies richest in potassium:

Mushrooms, 4 lg	415 mg
Broccoli, 5″ stalk, raw	380 mg
Tomatoes, 1 med	365 mg
Carrots, 1 lg	340 mg

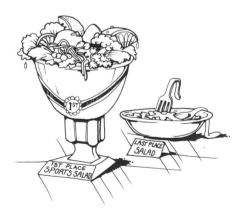

4.   For a meal-in-one salad, boost the protein value by adding flaked tuna, canned salmon, sliced turkey, chicken, or other lean meats. But be cautious of cold cuts and cheeses because they can add excess, saturated fat. Vegetarian proteins include diced tofu, chick-

peas (garbanzo beans), three-bean salad, walnuts, sunflower seeds, almonds, and peanuts.

Do remember that protein is an important part of a sports diet. Too often I counsel athletes who are so busy munching on salad greens and eating carbohydrates that they neglect their protein needs. They often end up anemic, injured, and chronically sick with colds or the flu (see chapter 9).

5. For calcium (and protein), add grated part-skim mozarella cheese, dressing made from plain yogurt seasoned with oregano, basil, and other Italian herbs, and/or a scoopful of low-fat cottage cheese (a better source of protein than of calcium). Drink low-fat milk (either skim, 1%, or 2%) along with the salad or have a fruit-flavored yogurt for dessert. Do be sure to get a calcium-rich, well-balanced salad if salads are the mainstay of your diet. Don't try to live on greens alone!

Salad Dressings

Salad dressings are an athlete's nemesis because they appease the appetite with fats rather than fuel the muscles with carbohydrates. A few ladles of blue cheese dressing can drown a small salad's healthfulness in 400 calories of fat. On a large salad, dressing can easily add 800 to 1,000 calories. But there are low-calorie and low-fat brands available with increasing frequency. Try to use them if you want to reduce your fat intake.

If you want to gain weight, generous amounts of olive oil (a heart-healthy fat) can easily boost your calorie intake. However, if you want to lose weight, these calories can devastate a diet. Salad dressing caused one wrestler to *gain* weight on his so-called reducing diet. When he traded in his supposedly fattening sandwich for a diet salad, he smothered his good intentions in 500 calories of oil. He would have been better off eating the sandwich or else using less oil and more calorie-free vinegar.

I often advise my clients to educate themselves about salad dressing calories by measuring out the amount of dressing they normally use on a salad and adjusting it according to their nutrition game plan. Refer to Table 5.2 for information about the calories in some popular dressings.

To reduce your intake of oily dressing calories, dilute dressings with vinegar, lemon juice, water, or milk. By using only small amounts of this diluted version, you'll get lots of flavor and moistness with fewer calories. Put the dressing in a bottle with a shaker top so that it comes out slowly, or even try putting it in a spray bottle. At restaurants, always request that the dressing be served on the side so that

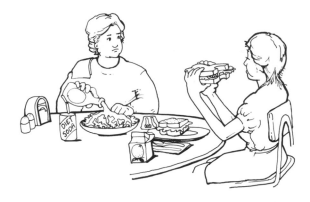

Table 5.2   Salad Dressing Calories

A few innocent ladles of salad dressing can transform a potentially healthful salad into a high-fat nutritional nightmare. Even "lite" dressings have calories—use them sparingly!

Dressing	Calories in 2 tablespoons	% Calories from fat
French	175	100
Oil and vinegar	140	100
Blue cheese	150	95
Caesar	140	90
"Lite" brands	30-70	50-90
Plain vinegar	5	—
Herbs, sprinkling	5	—

you can control the amount that you consume. Add the dressing sparingly; the calories accumulate quickly.

Low-calorie dressings are another alternative. But be forewarned—even "diet dressings" have calories in them and should be used sparingly. At home you might want to create your own low-calorie, creamy dressing by adding a little blue cheese or Italian seasonings to plain, low-fat yogurt. Or adventure into the world of exotic vinegars. Balsamic is one of my favorites.

By replacing these fat calories with more carbohydrates—an extra dinner roll or baked potato, or even sherbet for dessert—you can improve your body's capacity for exercise.

CHAPTER 6

Healthy Meals: At Home, on the Road, and on the Run

If you're like many of my clients, you arrive home after a hard work-out, devour the handiest food in sight, and then feel angry with your-self for having eaten junk instead of a wholesome dinner. Or, you get sidetracked into restaurants because you're too tired and hungry to cook. Restaurant eating, although expensive, can be a tempting alternative to confronting your own kitchen!

Athletes often come to me disgusted with themselves. They know they should be eating nutritiously, but they routinely raid the ice cream, munch out on pretzels, seek out the closest burger house, or dine on the handiest calories, opting for a "quick fix" rather than wholesome foods.

Dining In

The following tips will help you plan better sports meals at home. Even noncooks can pull together a high-carbohydrate, low-fat sports dinner without much time or effort. The recipes in Section IV offer tried and true suggestions. Here are some additional tips.

Tip #1: Prevent Yourself From Arriving Home TOO Hungry

One prerequisite to successful nighttime dining is to eat a hearty lunch or afternoon snack. As I explained in chapters 3 and 4, this prevents you from attacking the refrigerator the minute you walk in the house in the evening. Jack, a triathlete, felt both frustration and a sense of failure because he rarely had energy to prepare a nice dinner. "It's generally 8 or 9 o'clock by the time I finish my evening workout. At that point, I'm too famished to cook a well-balanced meal. I simply munch on whatever's around. Some days this means a box of crackers. Other days, it's a bag of chips. I know this is bad, but I'm just too hungry to care."

I found a very simple solution to Jack's problem: Eat a bigger meal at lunchtime rather than wait until evening. At that point in his day, he has easy access to good food in the cafeteria, he has time to eat, and he could save himself the hassle of cooking at night by swapping dinner with lunch.

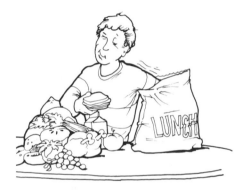

In one day, Jack discovered that the hearty noontime meal contributed not only to a higher quality evening workout but also to the presence of mind to prepare a more nourishing dinner.

Other people have alleviated the I'm-too-hungry-to-cook problem by simply eating a substantial afternoon snack. A 4 o'clock yogurt snack can prevent a 6 o'clock ice cream dinner.

Tip #2: Plan Time to Food Shop

Stock your kitchen shelves and freezer with a variety of wholesome foods that have a long shelf life. You're more likely to eat a better dinner if these nutritious choices are ready and waiting. For example, Kirsten, a 24-year-old dental assistant and swimmer, used to spend most of her food budget in restaurants on the way home from work because at home she faced bare cupboards and an empty refrigerator. Although she liked to cook, she rarely did so because she simply didn't plan the time to grocery shop. "Anyway, my schedule is so unpredictable. I often dine out with friends on the spur of the moment. When I do stock up on groceries, the meats and vegetables generally spoil before I get around to cooking them.''

I advised Kirsten to stock up on frozen vegetables—particularly vitamin-rich broccoli, spinach, and winter squash. Freezing does not destroy their nutritional value, so these veggies provide quick nutrition with less fuss or waste than with fresh produce. The frozen broccoli provides far more nutrients than the wilted, 5-day-old stalks that Kirsten occasionally dragged from her refrigerator.

Once she had stocked her kitchen with frozen veggies and other staples, Kirsten discovered that she liked to come home for dinner. Her staples included these items:

Carbohydrates

- Pasta, rice, noodles, and potatoes. Kirsten got into the habit of cooking double batches of rice or pasta. She stored the extra serving in a plastic bag and could reheat it quickly the next day by plunging it into boiling water for a minute. She reheated baked potatoes in the microwave.
- Whole grain crackers and breads. Kirsten stored the bread in the freezer and quickly thawed it in the toaster.
- Hot and cold cereals for a nontraditional dinner.

Vegetables and Fruits

- Frozen broccoli, spinach, and winter squash.
- Spaghetti sauce for pasta or for English muffin pizzas.
- Tomato and vegetable juice.
- Frozen orange juice.

Protein

- Canned clams, to toss into pasta. Clams are not only easy to fix, but they are also a great source of zinc. This mineral, important for healing, had been lacking in Kirsten's semivegetarian diet.
- Canned fish, for handy, no-cook meals. Tuna sandwiches, salmon on stoned-wheat crackers, and sardines with toast provided not only protein and iron but also the health-protective omega-3 fatty acids.

Dairy Products

- Part-skim mozzarella cheese, low-fat cottage cheese, yogurt, and nonfat milk powder. Kirsten could eat low-fat cheese, wheat crackers, and V-8 juice for a well-balanced but lazy meal when she had no desire to cook; or, she could top off a microwaved potato with low-fat cottage cheese or mix yogurt with muesli for a main course or dessert.

The adjacent chart lists some of the foods that I keep on hand along with menu suggestions using these staples.

Tip #3: Plan Cook-a-thons

Laura, a 48-year-old tennis player and stockbroker, enjoyed cooking on the weekends when she had the time.

She religiously created a big batch of something on Sunday so that it would be waiting for her when she arrived home tired and hungry after work and workouts. She preferred convenience to variety and thrived well on chili, chili, chili for a week; then curry, curry, curry the next week; goulash, goulash, goulash, and so on. When Laura couldn't face another repetitious dinner, she cooked something else and put the leftovers in the freezer. She preferred this monotonous but nutritious alternative to her previous habit of dining on ice cream by the pint.

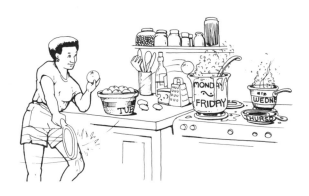

Dining Out

Some people enjoy eating in restaurants; others eat in restaurants because they have no choice. Art, a 54-year-old runner and businessman, yearns for homecooked meals, but due to the nature of his work he spends most of his evenings entertaining clients in the finest restaur-

Stocking Up on Good Nutrition

I always stock basic foods that won't spoil quickly. On days when I arrive home to an empty refrigerator, I can either pull together a noncooked meal or quickly prepare a hot dinner. Some of my standard menus include English muffin pizzas; stoned-wheat crackers, peanut butter, and milk; vegetable soup with extra broccoli and a sprinkling of parmesan; tuna sandwich with tomato soup; or bran cereal with banana and raisins.

My standard ingredients:

Cupboard	*Refrigerator*	*Freezer*
Spaghetti	"Lite" cheese	English muffins
Rice	Parmesan cheese	Pita bread
Ramen noodles	Low-fat cottage cheese	Multigrain bread
Potatoes	Low-fat yogurt	Orange juice concentrate
Wheat crackers	Low-fat milk	Broccoli
Ry-Krisp	Eggs	Spinach
Spaghetti sauce	Bananas	Winter squash
Minced clams	Carrots	Cut-up chicken
Tuna	V-8 juice	Extra-lean hamburger
Canned salmon		Ground turkey
Kidney beans		
Peanut butter		
Bran flakes		
Oat bran		
Muesli		
Raisins		

When creating a dinner from these staples, I choose items from three of the four food groups. The following are sample 650-calorie, 60-percent-carbohydrate, well-balanced meals—with no cooking!

Menu	Grain	Protein	Fruit/ Vegetable	Dairy
Crackers with salmon	8 stoned-wheat crackers	1/2 c canned salmon	12 oz V-8 juice	1 c fruit yogurt
Sandwhich	2 sl branola bread	2 T peanut butter	1/4 c raisins	1 c low-fat milk
Pizza	2 English muffins	(cheese)	3/4 c spaghetti sauce; 1 c orange juice	2 oz mozzarella cheese

The portions are appropriate for an active woman who needs about 1,800 to 2,000 calories per day; a hungry man may want more.

ants. Professional teams, such as the Boston Celtics, who travel from city to city often struggle with restaurant eating. After a hard evening game, the players may want nothing more than a friendly homecooked meal, but instead are often stuck in a hotel, challenged to find some healthy food at late hours of the night. Between jet lag, irregular meals, and night games, they have a tough struggle to find a high-carbohydrate sports diet that fuels and refuels their muscles for repeated hard exercise.

Traveling athletes also have the second challenge of keeping themselves well hydrated. Carrying a personal water supply is a good idea—particularly on planes, where the environment is very dry and water availability is somewhat limited.

Every sports-active person who relies on restaurants for a balanced high-carbohydrate diet faces the challenge of finding adequate carbohydrates among all the rich temptations, and each has pestered waiters for special requests at one time or another. Unfortunately, many people select whatever's fast and happens to tempt their tastebuds at the moment, particularly when they are tired, hungry, stressed, anxious, or lonely.

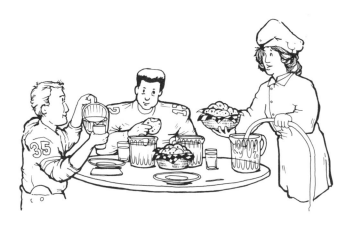

Here are a few suggestions for successfully selecting high-carbohydrate, low-fat restaurant meals with plenty of fluids. The most important first step is to patronize the restaurants that offer healthful sports foods; don't go to a steak house if you're looking for spaghetti! Study the menu before you sit down to see if the restaurant offers pasta, baked potatoes, bread, juices, and other high-carbohydrate items. Try to avoid the places that have only fried items. Also check to see if they allow special requests. If the menu clearly states "No Substitutions," you might be in the wrong place.

Once in an appropriate restaurant, choose your foods wisely. In general, you should request foods that are baked, broiled, roasted, or steamed—anything but fried. Low-fat poultry and fish items tend to be better choices than items naturally high in fat, such as prime rib, cheese, sausage, and duck.

Low-fat and Healthful Choices

Keep the following foods in mind as you peruse a menu.

Appetizers. Tomato juice, fruit juice, fruit cocktail, melon, and crackers.

Breads. Unbuttered rolls and breads are great—ask for extras! If the standard fare is buttered (as in garlic bread) request some plain bread also, and enjoy the buttery bread in moderation.

Soups. Broth-based soups (such as vegetable, chicken and rice, and Chinese soups and hearty minestrone, split pea, navy bean, and lentil soups can be good sources of carbohydrates and are preferable to creamy chowders and bisques. They're also good fluid sources.

Salads. Enjoy the veggies, but limit the creamed cottage cheese, bacon bits, grated cheese, olives, and other high-fat toppings. Be extra generous with chick-peas (garbanzo beans) and toasted croutons.

Salad Dressing. Always request that the dressing be served on the side so you can control how much you use. You want to fill up on carbohydrates, not oily dressings. (For additional information on salads, see chapter 5.)

Seafood and Poultry. Request chicken or fish that's baked, roasted, steamed, or broiled. Because many chefs add a lot of butter when broiling foods such as fish, you might want to request that your entrée be broiled dry—that is, cooked without this extra fat. If the entrée is sautéed, request that the chef sautée it with very little butter or oil and add no extra fat before serving.

Beef. Most restaurants pride themselves on serving huge slabs of beef or one-pound steaks. If you order beef, plan to cut this double portion in half and either take the rest home for tomorrow's dinner, share it with a companion (who has ordered accordingly), or simply leave it. Trim all the visible fat, and request that any gravy or sauces be served on the side so that you can use them sparingly, if at all. Your goal is to eat meat as the accompaniment to the meal, not as the focus. Your muscles will perform better if you fuel them with more carbohydrate-rich potatoes, vegetables, breads, and juices.

Potatoes.   Order extra to make this the mainstay of your dinner! Baked potatoes are a great source of carbohydrates, unless the chef loads them up with butter or sour cream. Request that these toppings be put on the side so that you can control how much you eat. Better yet, trade those fat calories for more carbohydrates. Add moistness by mashing the potato with some milk (special request). This may sound a bit messy, but it's a delicious, low-fat way to enjoy what might be an otherwise dry potato.

Pasta.   Pile it on! Pick pasta served with tomato sauces (carbohydrates) rather than the high-fat cheese, oil, or cream sauces.

Rice.   Another good source of carbohydrates. In a Chinese restaurant, you'll be better off filling up on an extra bowl of plain rice than eggrolls or other greasy appetizers.

Vegetables.   Request plain, unbuttered veggies with any special sauces (hollandaise, lemon butter) served on the side.

Chinese Food.   Plain rice with stir-fry combinations (such as chicken with veggies, beef with broccoli) are the best choices. You can request that the food be cooked with very little oil.

Dessert.   Sherbet and fruit are the highest carbohydrate choices. Fresh fruit is often available, even if it isn't listed on the menu. If you can't resist a dessert monstrosity, just be sure that you enjoy it *after* you eat plenty of carbohydrates. That is, don't have a carbohydrate-poor dinner to save room for a high-fat dessert.

Water.   Request a pitcher for the table so you can have endless refills without being a pest.

Beverages. Order double servings. Both juice and soft drinks are high-carbohydrate choices. Obviously, juice is nutritionally preferable to the empty calories in a soda pop, but both will fuel your muscles. Diet sodas provide only fluid, no fuel, low-fat milk is always a healthful choice.

The following list will help you choose high-carbohydrate dishes in ethnic restaurants.

International Carbohydrates

When it comes to carbohydrates, enjoy Chinese or Mexican as an alternative to the traditional Italian pasta.

Carbohydrates Chinese-style

Tips:

1. Special-request that your food be either steamed or stir-fried with minimal oil.
2. Order extra servings of rice, pancakes (that come with moo shi dishes), lo mein (noodles), or steamed buns.
3. Choose stir-fried rather than deep-fried items (often described as "crispy" or "dipped in batter").
4. Limit oily-looking sauces. Sweet and sour sauce is fine—just request it on stir-fried rather than deep-fried dishes.

Sample high-carbohydrate meals:

Menu #1
Egg drop soup
Chicken chop suey
Rice, boiled (double serving)
Fortune cookies

Menu #2
Wonton soup
Spicy orange chicken
Plain lo-mein noodles
  (special request)
Pineapple chunks

Carbohydrates Mexican-style

Tips:

1. Carbohydrate-rich choices include rice, beans, tortillas, and bean soups.
2. Request plain (*not* fried) tortillas with tostados.
3. Request reduced cheese in enchiladas, tacos, and other entrees, when possible.
4. Bean dishes are sometimes loaded with lard—be cautious!

Sample high-carbohydrate meals:

Menu #1
Bean burrito
Rice, large serving
Tortilla chips (only a few!)
Salsa

Menu #2
Chili
Rice
Corn tortillas (not fried)

Menu #3
Lime soup
Chicken enchilada
Beans and rice
Plain tortillas

When you're faced with a meal that's all wrong for you, try to make the best of a tough situation. For example, you can scoop the sour cream off the potato, drain the dressing from the salad, scrape off the gravy, or remove the fried batter from the chicken.

You can also top off a carbohydrate-poor meal with your own high-carbohydrate after-dinner snacks, such as fig bars, a muffin, pretzels, animal crackers, a banana, graham crackers, dried pineapple, raisins, and juice boxes. Pack these emergency foods along with you. However, also try to make special requests. Remember—*you* are the boss when it comes to restaurant eating. The restaurant's job is to serve you the high-carbohydrate, low-fat foods that enhance your sports diet. Bon appetit!

Fast Foods

Every day, one out of five Americans takes advantage of the convenience offered by fast-food restaurants. The omnipotence of the fast-food industry has even led some kids to think that the basic four food groups are McDonalds, Wendy's, Pizza Hut, and Kentucky Fried Chicken! Unfortunately, fast foods tend to offer proportionately more empty calories than wholesome goodness. If fast foods are a part of your lifestyle, you should at least learn how to make the best choices and eat them in good health.

Five Basic Faults

When you eat at a fast-food restaurant, you have an easy opportunity to select a dietary disaster. Here are the five basic faults to overcome:

1.   Fast foods are typically fat foods loaded with grease and saturated fats (see Table 6.1). A typical purchase of a burger, fries, and
a shake contains more than 1,100 calories of which 42 percent are from
fat and 45 percent are from carbohydrates. The fat is mostly saturated (even in the french fries) and these carbos are mostly refined sugar
and flour—less than wholesome.

2.   Fast foods generally lack the fiber found in more wholesome
foods. Burgers, chicken, and other animal products have no fiber, and
the bread and rolls that accompany them are usually made from refined flours.

Table 6.1   Fat and Salt in Fast Foods

A health-promoting sports diet provides less than 25 percent of calories from fat
and about 3,000 to 5,000 milligrams of sodium per day (2,000 to 3,000 milligrams
for those with high blood pressure). One fast-food meal can easily exceed those
targets, so counterbalance at the other meals that day.

	Total calories	% Calories from fat	Sodium (mg)
McDonald's			
Big Mac	565	55	1,010
Filet-o-fish	430	52	780
McNuggets	315	55	525
(6 pieces, no sauce)			
Wendy's			
Single burger	470	50	775
Double burger	670	55	980
Chocolate shake	390	37	250
Burger King			
Whopper with cheese	740	55	1,435
Onion rings, regular	270	55	450
Fries, regular	210	50	230
Kentucky Fried Chicken			
Original recipe dinner	640	50	1,440
Side breast, extra			
crispy	285	55	565

Note. Nutrient data from *Bowes and Church's Food Values of Portions Commonly Used*
(14th ed.) by J. Pennington and H. Church, 1985, Philadelphia: Lippincott.
Adapted by permission.

3.   Fast foods may be low in nutrients, especially vitamins A and C, unless you eat from a salad bar filled with fresh fruits and vegetables. Prepared fast-food salads are nothing to brag about either because they contain mostly pale lettuces that offer little nutritional value. Remember, too, that the salad dressings can add nearly 400 calories of fat!

4.   Fast foods are high in salt, which means they are high in sodium. Those special sauces and seasonings will spice up the flavor, but the extra sodium they contain may be a detriment. If you have high blood pressure, one meal can almost use up your day's allotment. For example, a Big Mac and fries has 1,100 milligrams of sodium. Physicians recommend that total daily intake not exceed 2,000 to 3,000 milligrams—just over 1 teaspoon—of sodium for blood pressure control (see Table 6.1).

5.   Fast-food fluids are usually sugar-laden soft drinks with zero vitamins and minerals or fat-filled shakes with limited nutritional benefits.

If you find yourself succumbing once in a while to any or all of these faults, then simply remember to balance out your day's remaining meals with wholesome, nutritious choices.

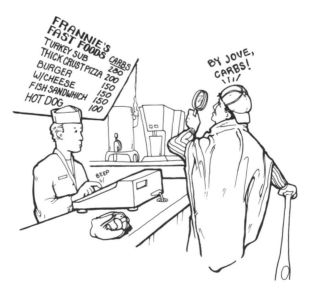

Fast-Food Carbohydrates

Although fast foods are usually pretty greasy, you *can* eat adequate carbohydrates at fast-food places, particularly if you supplement your meals with juice or fruit from the corner market. Here are some options:

Breakfast

- Rather than egg, bacon, sausage and/or croissant combinations, choose pancakes, hot or cold cereal, orange juice, and/or unbuttered biscuits, bagels, and muffins with jam.
- Because fruit can be hard to find on the menu, remember to carry some with you.
- Treat yourself to hot cocoa sometimes for a higher carbohydrate choice than coffee.
- If you're staying at a hotel, save yourself time, money, and temptations by bringing your own cereal and raisins (and spoon). Either mix-up powdered milk or buy a half-pint low-fat milk at the corner store. A water glass or milk carton can double as a cereal bowl.

Lunch and Dinner

- Burgers, fried chicken, and french fries all have a high fat content. You'll get more carbohydrates by sticking to the salad bar, a baked potato, and chili.
- If you do order a burger, request a second roll. Replace the greasy bottom half of the hamburger bun with half of the extra bun. Eat the other extra half plain.
- If you order fried chicken, get the larger pieces, remove all the skin, and eat just the meat. Order extra rolls, biscuits, or corn on the cob for more carbohydrates.
- At the salad bar, be generous with the colorful vegetables and hearty breads, but be careful not to overdose on oily dressings (see chapter 5 for more salad information).
- Resist the temptation to smother baked potatoes with cheese sauce and high-fat toppings. Wendy's cheese-stuffed potato, for example, gets 52 percent of its calories from fat (the equivalent of 9 teaspoons of butter).
- Order pizza with extra crust rather than extra cheese. The more dough, the more carbohydrates. Pile on veggies (green peppers, mushrooms, onions) but skip the pepperoni, sausage, and hamburger.
- Seek out a deli that offers wholesome breads. Request a sandwich that emphasizes the bread rather than the filling. "Hold the mayo" and add moistness with mustard or ketchup, sliced tomatoes, and lettuce.
- Hearty bean soups accompanied by crackers, plain bread, an English muffin, or a corn muffin provides a satisfying, carbohydrate-rich low-fat meal.

You can eat a high-carbohydrate sports diet, even if you're eating fast foods. You simply need to creatively balance the fats with the carbohydrates. For menu suggestions, see Table 6.2.

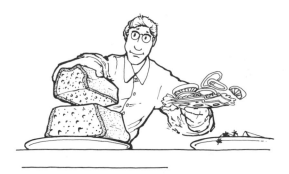

Table 6.2 Sample High Carbohydrate Fast Food Meals

The optimal sports diet gets 60 to 70 percent of its calories from carbohydrates. At fast-food restaurants, you can very easily consume a suboptimal 40 to 50 percent carbohydrate diet because fatty foods are readily available, inexpensive, and often tempting. You have to plan ahead. Bring wholesome snacks with you and make special requests when possible.

The menus below are sample sports meals that offer at least 60 percent carbohydrates. Some of the food items (such as soft drinks and milk shakes) are not generally recommended as a part of an optimal daily diet, but they can be part of a meal-on-the-road from time to time. The purpose of these sample meals is simply to give you an idea of what a 60 percent carbohydrate diet looks like, so that you can use this to guide your food choices. The menus are appropriate for active women and men who need 2,000 to 2,600+ calories per day. *For extra carbohydrates, eat more of the foods in italics.*

Meal	Item	Total calories
Breakfast		
McDonald's/Fast Foods:	*Orange juice,* 6 oz	85
	Pancakes, syrup	420
	English muffin, jelly	155
Total: 85% carbohydrates; 660 calories		
Muffin House Bakery	*Bran muffin,* lg	320
	Hot cocoa, lg	180
Total: 60% carbohydrates; 500 calories		
Family restaurant	*Apple juice,* lg	145
	Raisin Bran, 2 sm boxes	220
	Low-fat milk, 8 oz	110
	Sliced banana, med	125
Total: 92% carbohydrates; 590 calories		

Meal	Item	Total calories

Lunch

Sub shop	Turkey sub, no mayo	655
	Fruit yogurt	260
	Orange juice, half-pint	110

Total: 63% carbohydrates; 1,025 calories

Wendy's/Fast Food:	*Plain baked potato*	240
	Chili, 1 c	230
	Chocolate shake	390

Total: 60% carbohydrates; 1,025 calories

Salad bar:	Lettuce, 1 c	15
	Green pepper, 1/2	10
	Broccoli, 1/2 c	20
	Carrots, 1/2 c	20
	Tomato, lg	50
	Chick-peas, 1/2 c	170
	Feta cheese, 1 oz	75
	Italian dressing, 2 T	100
	Bread, 1" sl	200

Total: 60% carbohydrates; 660 calories

Dinner

Pizza:	Cheese pizza, 4 sl, 13"	920
	Large cola, 12 oz	150

Total: 63% carbohydrates; 1,070 calories

Italian restaurant:	Minestrone soup, 1 c	85
	Spaghetti, 2 c	400
	Tomato sauce, 2/3 c	120
	Parmesan cheese, 1 T	30
	Rolls, 2 lg	280

Total: 74% carbohydrates; 915 calories

Family restaurant:	Turkey, 5 oz white meat	250
	Stuffing, 1 c	200
	Mashed potato, 1/2 c	95
	Peas, 2/3 c	70
	Cranberry sauce, 1/4 c	100
	Orange juice, 8 oz	110
	Sherbet, 1 scoop	120

Total: 64% carbohydrates; 945 calories

Sports Nutrition

The Science of Eating for Success

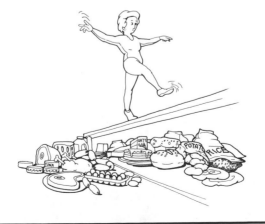

CHAPTER 7

Carbohydrates: Simplifying a Complex Issue

Without question, carbohydrates are the best choice for fueling your muscles and promoting the health of your heart. People of all ages and athletic abilities, from elite runners to spectators, should nourish themselves with a wholesome, high-carbohydrate, low-fat sports diet.

Unfortunately, misconceptions about carbohydrates—what they are and what they aren't—keep many people from making good carbohydrate selections. As one runner put it, "I know I should eat carbohydrates for muscle fuel, but which are best? Does it matter if I choose fruits, vegetables, sugar, refined flour, or brown rice?" Like many active people, he was confused by this seemingly complex subject.

The purpose of this chapter is to eliminate this confusion so you can make choices that best promote your health, desired weight, and performance.

Simple Sugars

The carbohydrate family includes both simple and complex carbohydrates. The simple ones are *monosaccharides* and *disaccharides* (single and double sugar molecules). Glucose, fructose, and galactose are the simplest sugars and can be symbolized like this:

The disaccharides can be symbolized like this:

Two common disaccharides include table sugar (sucrose—a combination of glucose and fructose) and milk sugar (lactose—a combination of glucose and galactose). These get converted into glucose molecules before entering into the bloodstream for fuel.

Table sugar and honey both contain glucose and fructose but in different forms. Table sugar is made of disaccharides that get converted to monosaccharides: 50 percent glucose and 50 percent fructose. Honey contains monosaccharides: 31 percent glucose, 38 percent fructose, 10 percent other sugars, 17 percent water, and 4 percent miscellaneous particles. Table 7.1 describes the types of sugars found in some fruits and vegetables.

Table 7.1 Natural Sugars in Some Fruits and Vegetables

Fruits and vegetables contain mixtures of different types of sugars. All sugars are converted into glucose before being used for energy.

Food	Glucose	Fructose	Sucrose
		(% of total solids)	
Apple	7	40	25
Grapes	35	40	12
Peaches	7	10	55
Carrots	7	7	35
Green beans	15	15	3
Tomato	20	25	—

Note. Data from *The Food That Stays: An Update on Nutrition, Diet, Sugar and Calories* by E. Sweeney (Ed.), 1977, American Academy of Pediatrics. New York: Med Com, Inc.

Some athletes mistakenly think that honey is nutritionally superior to refined white sugar. If you prefer honey because of the pleasant taste, fine. But it's not superior for health or performance. Sugar in any form—honey, brown sugar, raw sugar, maple syrup, or jelly—

Table 7.2 Nutritional Value of Sugar

Although natural sugars may have a bit more nutritional value than refined white sugar, no sugars are significant sources of vitamins or minerals.

	Calories (per T)	Calcium (mg)	Iron (mg)	Riboflavin (mg)
White	46	trace	—	—
Brown	52	11	0.4	—
Honey	61	1	1.0	.01
RDA	—	800	18	1.8

Note. Nutrient data from *Bowes and Church's Food Values of Portions Commonly Used* (14th ed.) by J. Pennington and H. Church, 1985, Philadelphia: Lippincott. Adapted by permission.

has insignificant amounts of vitamins or minerals. Table 7.2 compares the nutritional value of some sugars.

A third type of sugar that has recently entered the sports market is the *glucose polymer*. Polymers are chains of about five glucose molecules. Sports drinks sweetened with polymers can provide more energy value with less sweetness than sugar. Chapter 10 further addresses this issue.

Your body digests any type of sugar or carbohydrate into glucose before using it for fuel. Your muscles and brain require blood glucose for energy. The muscles can store glucose and burn fat; the brain does neither. Hence, adequate sugar from the blood is essential for the brain to function optimally. Athletes with low blood sugar tend to perform poorly because the poorly fueled brain limits muscular function and mental drive.

Complex Carbohydrates

Complex carbohydrates, such as starch in plant foods and glycogen in muscles, are formed when sugars link together to form long, complex chains, similar to a string of hundreds of pearls. They can be symbolized like this:

Plants store extra sugars in the form of starch. For example, corn on the cob, which is sweet when it's young, becomes starchy as it gets older. Its extra sugar converts into starch. In contrast to corn and other vegetables, fruits tend to convert starches into sugars as they ripen. A familiar example is the banana: A green banana with some yellow is 80 percent starch and 7 percent sugar; a mainly yellow banana is 25 percent starch and 65 percent sugar; a spotted and speckled banana is 5 percent starch and 90 percent sugar.

The potatoes, rice, bread, and other starches that you eat are digested into glucose, then either burned for energy or stored for future use (see the illustration). Humans all store extra dietary sugars in the form of *muscle glycogen* and *liver glycogen*. This glycogen is readily available for energy during exercise.

Sugars and starches have similar abilities to fuel muscles but different abilities to nourish them with vitamins and minerals:

- The carbohydrates in sugary soda pop provide energy but no vitamins or minerals.
- The carbohydrates in polymer drinks provide energy but no vitamins or minerals, unless the drink is fortified.
- The carbohydrates in wholesome fruits, vegetables, and grains provide energy, vitamins, and minerals—the fuel and spark plugs that your engine needs to function at its best.

Glucose and Glycogen

The average 150-pound active male has about 1,800 calories of carbohydrates stored in his liver, muscles, and blood in approximately the following distribution:

Muscle glycogen	1,400 cal
Liver glycogen	320 cal
Blood glucose	80 cal
Total:	1,800 cal

These carbohydrate stores determine how long you can exercise. When you run out of glycogen, you hit the wall—that is, you feel overwhelmingly fatigued and yearn to quit.

In comparison to the approximately 1,800 calories of stored carbohydrates, the average *lean* 150-pound man also has about 60,000 to 100,000 calories of stored fat—enough to run hundreds of miles! Unfortunately for endurance athletes, fat cannot be used exclusively as fuel because the muscles need a certain amount of carbohydrates to function well; carbohydrates are a limiting factor for endurance athletes.

Steps of Digestion: Food into Fuel

The digestive tract is like a processing plant, breaking down complex foods containing carbohydrates, proteins, and fats into the more usable products—glucose, amino acids, and fatty acids.

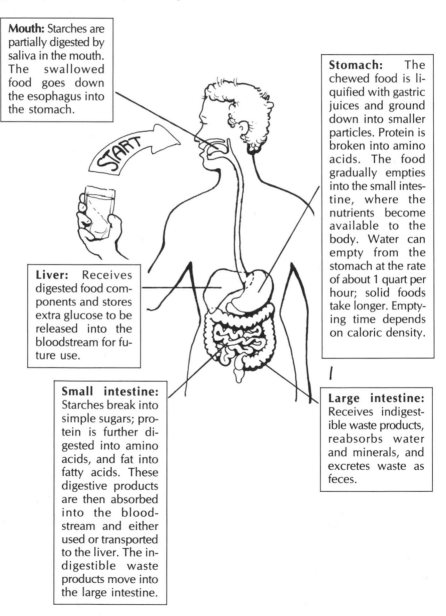

Mouth: Starches are partially digested by saliva in the mouth. The swallowed food goes down the esophagus into the stomach.

Stomach: The chewed food is liquified with gastric juices and ground down into smaller particles. Protein is broken into amino acids. The food gradually empties into the small intestine, where the nutrients become available to the body. Water can empty from the stomach at the rate of about 1 quart per hour; solid foods take longer. Emptying time depends on caloric density.

Liver: Receives digested food components and stores extra glucose to be released into the bloodstream for future use.

Small intestine: Starches break into simple sugars; protein is further digested into amino acids, and fat into fatty acids. These digestive products are then absorbed into the bloodstream and either used or transported to the liver. The indigestible waste products move into the large intestine.

Large intestine: Receives indigestible waste products, reabsorbs water and minerals, and excretes waste as feces.

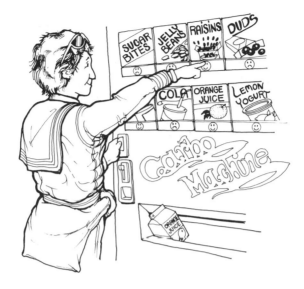

   During low-level exercise such as typing, the muscles burn primarily fats for energy. During light to moderate aerobic exercise, such as jogging, stored fat provides 50 to 60 percent of the fuel. When you exercise hard, as in sprinting or racing, you rely primarily on the glycogen stores.
   Biochemical changes that occur during training influence the amount of glycogen you can store in your muscles. Well-trained muscles develop the ability to store about 20 to 50 percent more glycogen than untrained muscles (Costill, 1979; Sherman, 1981). This enhances endurance capacity and is one reason why a novice runner can't simply carbo-load and run a top-quality marathon.

Muscle Glycogen per 100 g (3.5 oz) of muscle:

Untrained muscle:	13 g
Trained muscle:	32 g
Carbo-loaded muscle:	35–40 g

Bonking

Depleted *muscle* glycogen causes athletes to hit the wall; depleted *liver* glycogen causes them to "bonk" or "crash." Liver glycogen is fed into the bloodstream to maintain a normal blood sugar level essential for "brain food." Despite adequate muscle glycogen, an athlete may feel uncoordinated, light-headed, unable to concentrate, and weakened because the liver is releasing inadequate sugar into the bloodstream.

This happened to John, a 28-year-old runner and banker, at his first Boston Marathon. He had religiously carbo-loaded his muscles for 3 days prior to the event. On the evening before the marathon, he ate dinner at 5:00, then went to bed at 8:30 to ensure himself a good night's rest. But, as often happens with anxious athletes, he tossed and turned all night (which burned off a significant amount of calories), got up early the next morning, and chose not to eat breakfast, even though the marathon didn't start until noon. By noon, he had depleted his limited liver glycogen stores. He lost his mental drive about 8 miles into the race and quit at 12 miles. His muscles were well fueled, but that energy was unavailable to his brain so he lacked the mental stamina to endure the marathon.

John could have prevented this needless fatigue by eating some bread, cereal, or other carbohydrate at breakfast to refuel his liver glycogen stores. Athletic success depends on both well-fueled muscles *and* a well-fueled mind (see chapter 8 for more information).

Runners and Body Builders: Similar Diets?

"I've heard that for running I should eat carbohydrates to fuel my muscles. But for weight lifting, shouldn't I eat a lot of protein to build them up?"

Perhaps, like Julie, a 34-year-old runner who works out with Nautilus equipment, you're confused about what to eat for energy, strength, and top performance—carbohydrates or protein. I recommend this:

1. Eat carbohydrate-rich breakfasts, such as cereal rather than eggs.
2. Focus your lunches and dinners on breads, potatoes, pasta, rice, fruits, and vegetables. Two thirds of your plate should be covered with these carbohydrates.
3. Eat fish, chicken, lean meats, peanut butter, low-fat cheese, and other proteins as an accompaniment to meals—not as the main focus. Or eat carbohydrate-rich protein alternatives such as beans and rice, lentil soup, chili, and other vegetarian choices.

Carbohydrate is best because unlike protein and fat, it is readily stored in your muscles for fuel during exercise. Small amounts of protein are important for building and protecting your muscles, but you should dedicate only one third of your dinner plate to protein-rich foods. The rest should be carbohydrates (see chapter 9 for more about protein requirement).

Research by exercise physiologist Dr. J. Bergstrom (1967) explains why carbohydrates are essential for high-energy athletic performance. He compared the rate at which muscle glycogen was replaced in subjects who exercised to exhaustion and then ate either a high-protein, high-fat diet or a high-carbohydrate diet (Figure 7.1).

The subjects on the high protein, high-fat diet (similar to the diets of folks who live on steak, eggs, hamburger, tuna salad, peanut butter, and cheese) remained glycogen depleted for 5 days. The subjects on a high-carbohydrate diet totally replenished their muscle glycogen in 2 days. Conclusion: Proteins and fats don't get stored as muscle fuel; carbohydrates are the better source of energy.

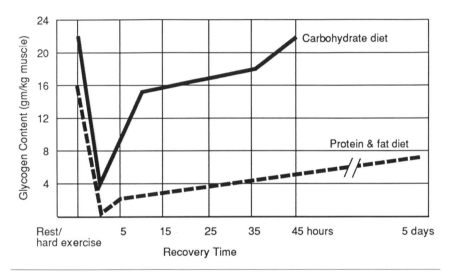

Figure 7.1. *Note:* From "Diet, Muscle Glycogen and Physical Performance" by J. Bergstrom, 1967, *Acta Physiologica Scandinavica,* **71**, p. 140. Copyright 1967 by *Acta Physiologica Scandinavica.* Reprinted by permission.

Carbohydrates for Daily Recovery

Carbohydrates are important not only for endurance athletes but also for those who train hard day after day and want to maintain high energy. If you want a low-carbohydrate diet, your muscles will feel chronically fatigued. You'll train, but not at your best.

Figure 7.2 shows the glycogen depletion that can occur when athletes eat an inadequate amount of carbohydrates and try to maintain an exercise routine (Costill, 1971). On 3 consecutive days, the subjects ran hard for 10 miles (at a pace of 6 to 8 minutes per mile). They ate their standard meals—a diet that provided about 45 to 50 percent of calories from carbohydrates, not the 60 to 65 percent required in

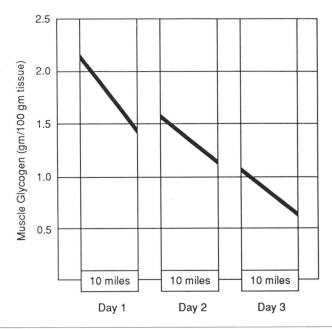

Figure 7.2. *Note:* From "Effect of Plasma FFA and Insulin on Muscle Glycogen Usage During Exercise" by D. Costill, E. Coyle, G. Dalsky et al. 1977, *Journal of Applied Physiology,* **43**, p. 695. Copyright 1977 by the American Physiological Society. Reprinted by permission.

a top-performance sports diet. The subjects' muscles became increasingly glycogen depleted, and subjects felt increasingly fatigued. Had they eaten larger portions of carbohydrates (and smaller portions of protein and fat), they would have replaced their glycogen stores better and performed better in the exercise tests.

This study emphasizes the need not only for a daily carbohydrate-rich diet but also for rest days with light or no training. The runners required extra rest time for their muscles to replace the burned-up glycogen. Depleted muscles need about 2 days to refuel after exhaustive exercise. An adequate recovery program is particularly important for endurance athletes because they deplete significantly more glycogen than the casual exerciser during their intense workouts.

Case in Point

Pat, a 33-year-old computer programmer and former compulsive runner, learned the importance of rest days and adequate carbohydrates through a sports nutrition experiment. She insisted on training every day to get in shape for the Boston Marathon. I invited her to vary her recovery diet to determine whether her running improved with running less and eating better.

Pat accepted the invitation and started to experiment with her 2-hour Sunday run.

Experiment #1.   After her workout, she ate her favorite brunch—a high-protein, high-fat, three-egg cheese omelette. When she ran on Monday, her legs were "dead"—tired, heavy, and unrecovered from hard effort.

Experiment #2.   The next Sunday, Pat ate a high-carbohydrate recovery meal: pancakes, maple syrup, orange juice, and fresh fruit. She ran on Monday and felt better than the previous week, but not great. She still needed more time to recover from Sunday's depleting workout.

Experiment #3.   The third Sunday, Pat ate the same breakfast as in Experiment #2, but she took a rest day on Monday. On Tuesday, she ran effortlessly. "I felt super—lots of energy, totally recovered, and ready for action. I haven't done a high-quality Tuesday workout like that for a long time."

Based on this experience, Pat concluded that a rest day for refueling after a hard workout was a worthwhile investment. She stopped forcing herself to do the obligatory daily training run on the days when her muscles felt fatigued. Instead, she planned at least one rest day per week into her training schedule and started doing quality, rather than quantity, training. Her running improved, as did her mental outlook and her enthusiasm for her sport. She ran a personal best in the marathon, cutting 8 minutes off her time.

Carbo-Loading for Endurance Events

When it comes to preparing for a marathon, triathlon, long-distance bike race, or other endurance event that will last for more than 90 minutes of intense exercise, you should

- reduce your training and rest your muscles to allow them to become saturated with carbohydrates, and
- eat a high-carbohydrate (60- to 70-percent) diet for 3 days prior to the event.

In times past, some athletes followed a week-long regimen involving an exhaustive bout of exercise followed by 3 depletion days of a low-carbohydrate diet, then 3 loading days of a high-carbohydrate intake. Recent research indicates that the depletion phase offers no performance benefits (Sherman, 1981).

Today exercise physiologists agree that the most effective way to prepare for a major endurance event is to eat a diet that is 60 to 70 percent carbohydrate while resting the muscles to allow them the chance to store the carbohydrates. For those athletes who eat a high-carbohydrate diet daily, the biggest change involves training less. In chapter 8, I provide more information about carbohydrate-loading.

Are Carbohydrates Fattening?

Some athletes eat too few carbohydrates because they believe them to be fattening. Jamie, a 17-year-old gymnast, wanted to eat carbohydrates for fuel yet also wanted to lose weight for gymnastics. Like many dieters, Jamie considered carbohydrates to be forbidden foods, and she was frustrated. "I don't keep crackers, bread, cereal, or bagels in the house because when they're there I eat them...too many of them! I want to lose weight, not gain it from those fattening carbohydrates."

After all, almost everyone knows that if you want to lose weight, you follow the advice of diet gurus who advise eating as much protein-rich foods as you want, but avoiding at all costs the sinful carbohydrates. Right?

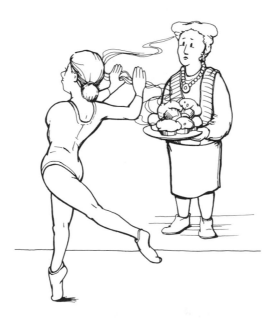

WRONG! Those diet gurus offer bad advice. Carbohydrates are not fattening! Fats are fattening—and many protein foods contain a lot of fat (cream in cheese, mayonnaise in tuna, grease in meat). Fats provide 36 calories per teaspoon, as compared to carbohydrates with 16.

Carbohydrates become fattening when you add hefty doses of fat, such as butter on bread and sour cream on potatoes. Due to this carbs-are-fattening misconception, many weight-conscious athletes report they're trying to stay away from carbohydrates.

Remember these points:

- Carbohydrates are not fattening.
- You need carbohydrates to fuel your muscles.
- You burn carbohydrates off during hard exercise.
- Carbohydrates are a friendly fuel; the "enemy" is too many fats.
- You should energize with cereal, bread, pasta, and potato, but limit your intake of the butter, margarine and mayonnaise that often accompany them.

See chapter 14 for more on weight reduction in carbohydrates.

All too often I talk to athletes who think they eat a carbohydrate-rich diet when they really don't. Jim, a 19-year-old college student, intended to carbo-load the night before the Newport Marathon with a pizza "supreme." Little did he know that of the 1,800 calories in the large pizza, 1,200 were from the protein and fat in the double cheese, sausage, and pepperoni. Only 35 percent of the calories from the thin crust and tomato sauce were carbohydrate. No wonder he felt sluggish during the race. Table 7.3 lists some other carbohydrates with hidden fats.

I gave Jim a list, *Carbohydrates Content of Commonly Eaten Foods* (Table 7.4), to post on his refrigerator. With this tool he learned to select high-carbohydrate foods.

In addition, I taught him how to make better selections based on food label information. You, too, should learn to use labels to guide your selections.

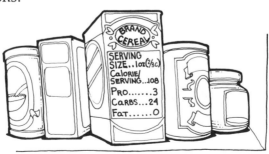

Table 7.3   Carbohydrates With Hidden Fats

Carbohydrates can be fattening if they have hidden fats. The following foods have fooled many unsuspicious athletes into thinking they're fueling up on carbohydrates when they're actually filling up on fats. Your target fat intake for the day should be about 25 percent of your total calories.

Food	% Calories from fat	Higher carbohydrate alternative	% Calories from fat
Croissant	60	Bagel, plain	5
Ritz crackers	50	Ak-Mok crackers	15
Pizza, thin crust	45	Pizza, thick crust	30
Coffee cake	45	Muffin, homemade	25
Macaroni and cheese	40	Pasta, tomato sauce	10
Granola	35	Grape-Nuts	1

Note. Nutrient data from *Bowes and Church's Food Values of Portions Commonly Used* (14th ed.) by J. Pennington and H. Church, 1985, Philadelphia: Lippincott. Adapted by permission.

Table 7.4   Carbohydrate Content of Commonly Eaten Foods

To fuel your muscles, you should try to get 60 to 70 percent of your calories from carbohydrates. If you need about 3,000 calories, 1,800 of them (60% × 3,000 = 1,800) should be from carbohydrates. There are 4 calories per gram of carbohydrate, so this translates into 450 grams—your target. The following list of carbohydrate-rich foods can help you keep a tally. Food labels are another handy source of carbohydrate information.

Food	Amount	Carbohydrates (g)	Total calories*
Fruits			
Apple	1 med	20	80
Orange	1 med	20	80
Banana	1 med	25	105
Raisins	1/4 c	30	120
Apricots, dried	8 hlvs	30	120
Fruit Roll-Up	2	24	100
Vegetables			
Corn, canned	1/2 c	18	80
Winter squash	1/2 c	15	65

Food	Amount	Carbohydrates (g)	Total calories*
Tomato sauce, Ragu	1/2 c	10	80
Peas	1/2 c	10	60
Carrot	1 med	10	40
Green beans	1/2 c	7	30
Broccoli	1 stalk	5	30
Zucchini	1/2 c	4	20
Bread-type foods			
Submarine roll	8″ lg	60	280
Branola bread, wheat	2 sl	35	210
Bagel, Lender's	1	30	160
English muffin, Thomas's	1	25	130
Pita pocket	1/2 of 8″round	22	120
Bran muffin	1 lg	45	320
Pancakes, Aunt Jemima	2 × 4″	30	140
Waffle, Eggo	1	17	120
Matzo	1 sheet	28	115
Saltines	6	15	90
Graham crackers	2 sq	11	60
Breakfast cereals			
Grape-Nuts	1/4 c	23	100
Raisin Bran	1/2 c	21	90
Granola	1/4 c	18	130
Oatmeal, maple instant	1 pkt	30	160
Cream of Wheat	1 svg	22	100
Beverages			
Apricot nectar	8 oz	35	140
Cranraspberry	8 oz	36	145
Apple	8 oz	30	120
Orange	8 oz	25	110
Gatorade	8 oz	10	40
Cola	12 oz	38	150
Beer	12 oz	13	150
Milk, chocolate	8 oz	25	150
Milk, low-fat 2%	8 oz	13	110
Grains, pasta, starches			
Baked potato	1 lg	55	240
Baked beans	1 c	50	330
Lentils, cooked	1 c	40	215

(Cont.)

Table 7.4 (Continued)

Food	Amount	Carbohydrates (g)	Total calories*
Stuffing	1 c	40	220
Spaghetti, cooked	1 c	40	200
Rice, cooked	1 c	35	160
Ramen noodles	1/2 pkg	25	200
Entrees, convenience foods			
Bean burrito	1	50	350
Chili	1 c	45	250
Macaroni and cheese	1 c	45	390
Pizza, cheese	2 sl	42	340
Big Mac	1	40	560
Split pea soup	11 oz	35	220
Chow mein	1 c	5	70
Sweets, snacks, desserts			
Maple syrup	2 T	25	100
Strawberry jam	1 T	13	50
Honey	1 T	15	60
Cranberry sauce	2 T	15	60
Fig Newtons	1	11	60
Chocolate chip cookie	1	10	65
Oreo	1	7	50
Poptart, blueberry	1	35	210
Fruit yogurt	1 c	50	260
Dairy Queen	1 med cone	35	230

*Includes calories from protein and fat

Note. Nutrient data from *Bowes and Church's Food Values of Portions Commonly Used* (14th ed.) by J. Pennington and H. Church, 1985, Philadelphia: Lippincott. Adapted by permission.

You should know that carbohydrate, protein, fat, and alcohol each have a specific number of calories per gram: Most food labels lists the number of grams of carbohydrate, protein, and fat (and alcohol, if present) per serving.

- 1 g carbohydrate = 4 cal
- 1 g protein = 4 cal
- 1 g fat = 9 cal
- 1 g alcohol = 7 cal

Now that you know the calories per gram, you can make some simple calculations. To determine the number of carbohydrate calories in a food item, multiply the number of grams of carbohydrate by 4 (calories per gram). Next, compare the carbohydrate calories to the total calories per serving to determine the percentage of calories that are from carbohydrates.

For example, ice cream (that all-time favorite "carbohydrate") contains fewer carbohydrates than you may realize. Ice milk, on the other hand has more.

- One-half cup of ice cream has about 15 grams of carbohydrate, which equals 60 calories of carbohydrate ($15 \times 4 = 60$). Since there are 170 total calories per 1/2 cup of ice cream, this means that only approximately 35 percent of the calories are from carbohydrates ($60 \div 170 = 35\%$).
- In comparison, 1/2 cup of ice milk contains 22 grams of carbohydrate, which equals 88 calories of carbohydrate ($22 \times 4 = 88$). Since there are 120 total calories per 1/2 cup of ice milk, this means that about 75 percent of the calories are from carbohydrates ($88 \div 120 \approx 75\%$).

Counting Carbohydrates

Your diet should be at least 60 percent carbohydrate for daily training, and 65 to 70 percent carbohydrate before an endurance event. You can achieve a diet that is 60 to 70 percent carbohydrate by opting for more starches and grains and fewer fatty, greasy foods: for instance, replacing croissants with bagels, eggs with pancakes, and steak with pasta. See Table 7.5 for additional examples.

Like many registered dietitians and sports nutritionists, I use a computer program that calculates the percentage of carbohydrate and fat in a diet so that athletes can see how their intake compares to the target goals of 60 percent carbohydrate, 25 percent fat, and 15 percent protein.

Dave, a 27-year-old nutrition fanatic, was flabbergasted to discover that his diet was only 50 percent carbohydrates. "I've been eating many more carbohydrates than I used to! And I really don't eat any extra fats. I've stopped using butter, mayonnaise, and salad dressing. Are you sure that your computer is working properly?"

The computer was fine. Dave simply indulged in too many peanuts, almonds, granola, and sunflower seeds—his favorite fat-filled snacks.

Table 7.5   Calculated Carbohydrates

When you are reading food labels, you can translate grams of fat and carbohydrate into percentage of calories.

- 1 g fat = 9 cal
- 1 g carbohydrate = 4 cal

This information will help you make the wisest choices for your sports diet. Be aware, however, that in some high-carbohydrate foods, such as fruit yogurt, the carbohydrates are from nutritionally empty sugar calories. Be sure to include adequate wholesome carbohydrates, not only refined sugars.

Food	Total calories	% Cals from carbohydrates (g)	% Cals from fat (g)
1 c blueberry yogurt, Dannon	260	75 (50)	10 (3)
1-3/4 c plain yogurt, Dannon	260	45 (30)	25 (7)
1-1/3 bran muffin, Duncan-Hines	260	68 (42)	30 (9)
1 chocolate croissant, Sara Lee	260	38 (25)	60 (17)
2/3 c split pea soup, Campbell's	200	60 (29)	20 (5)
1 c cream of mushroom soup, Campbell's	200	30 (18)	60 (14)
2 bagels, Lender's	300	80 (60)	5 (2)
1 bagel + 3 T cream cheese	300	40 (30)	50 (17)

Upon trading them in for higher carbohydrate items—pretzels, raisins, dried apricots, and bananas—he easily boosted his carbohydrate intake to 68 percent. "You know, my training has improved since I made that switch. My muscles seem to feel springier and have greater endurance. I feel great; I'm glad I learned this simple solution to my needless fatigue!"

If you want to feel in complete control of your diet and be sure that you're eating the right balance of carbohydrates, protein, and fat, have your diet evaluated by a computer. Or do it yourself by counting grams of carbohydrates, based on your body's needs. Here's how:

- The 60 percent target carbohydrate intake for an active woman who requires 2,000 calories is

60% x 2,000 cal = 1,200 carbohydrate cal

Divide this by 4 calories per gram of carbohydrate:

= 300 g carbohydrates/day

- For an active man who requires 3,500 calories, the 60 percent target carbohydrate intake is

60% x 3,500 cal = 2,100 carbohydrate cal

Divide this by 4 calories per gram of carbohydrate:

= 525 g carbohydrates/day.

I urge you to become an avid label reader and count the grams of carbohydrate you eat. This way, you'll learn more about your daily training diet to be sure that you're getting adequate carbohydrates. I generally see more athletes carbohydrate-depleted during training sessions than before competitions. They take good care of themselves prior to an important event but often neglect their training diets. Unfortunately they can't compete at their best if they don't train at their best.

Carbohydrates Versus Fats: A Delicate Balance

Although you want to maximize your intake of carbohydrates and minimize your intake of fats, you shouldn't cut out all fats from your sports diet. I overheard one runner advising her buddy, "Be sure to stay away from all fats before the race. Fatty foods prevent you from storing the glycogen in your muscles." This simply is false. Fat does not interfere with glycogen storage.

However, if you want to fuel your muscles, don't stuff yourself with too much fat, such as fettuccini alfredo's butter and cheese sauce, and so eat inadequate carbohydrates. You'll be better off eating pasta with carbohydrate-filled tomato sauce. After you have carbo-loaded, you can then splurge on dessert, if you like. The point is: First fuel up on carbohydrates, then (if you still have the yen), fill in the cracks with fats.

Another mistake common to dedicated athletes is reducing fat intake without replacing those calories with adequate carbohydrates.

Don, a basketball player, cut butter, mayonnaise, and salad dressing from his diet and lost 3 pounds within a week of this nutrition change; he neglected to replace the deleted fat calories with adequate carbohydrates. He should, for example, have eaten two potatoes to get the same amount of calories in the one potato drenched with butter and sour cream.

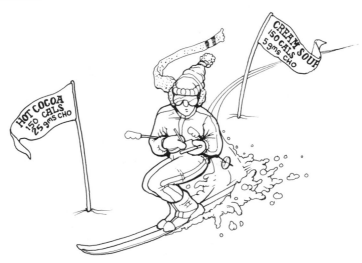

Athletes who choose very low-fat diets must eat large quantities of carbohydrates to get adequate calories. If they have big appetites, as do 6'10" basketball players, they often tire of chewing before they are adequately fed! The main focus of the diet should be on carbohydrates, but some fats can still be included. After all, about 25 percent of the calories in a sports diet are allotted to fat: 25% x 3,000 calories = 750 fat calories; divided by 9 calories per gram, this equals 83 grams of fat. Chapter 2 offers more information on appropriate fat intake.

In addition to counting grams of carbohydrate (as I suggested above), try counting grams of fat for a day or two. Select foods that have nutrition information on the labels, measure the portions, and tally the grams. Some simple meals based on foods with nutrition labeling might be cereal, milk, and juice; a peanut butter sandwich and yogurt; and soup and an english muffin with low-fat cheese. This educational experience can give you the peace of mind of knowing you're making wise choices that promote both health and performance.

CHAPTER 8

Nutrition Before Exercise: Pre-Event Foods

Every athlete wants to know what's best to eat before exercising. I only wish I had the winning recipe! The ingredients for the best pretraining or precompetition meal include both physiological and psychological factors. Each person has unique food preferences and aversions, so no one food or "magic meal" will ensure top performance for everyone. For example:

• Herbert, an elite marathon runner, thrives best on two slices of plain bread an hour before his morning run. "It absorbs the stomach juices and settles my stomach." He follows the same routine before he competes.

• Mary Ellen, a rugby player and secretary, avoids any food within 4 hours of training or competing. Otherwise she has horrible stomach cramps.

• Tim, a competitive cyclist, claims he *must* eat cereal. "My magic food is raisin bran with a banana. I've always had my best training rides and races after this breakfast."

• Tracy, a figure skater and 7th-grade student, snacks on a banana before practice sessions but on nothing before a competition. She gets so nervous that she can't keep anything down. "I try to make sure I eat extra good the day before a competition."

Choices of what to eat before exercising vary from person to person and from sport to sport with no single right or wrong choice. My experience has shown that each athlete has to learn through trial and error during training and competitions what works best for his or her body—and what doesn't work. Some athletes can eat almost anything; others want special foods. And then there are the "abstainers" who have absolutely no desire to eat anything. All can perform superbly.

Athletes in running sports, where the body moves up and down, tend to abstain from food more than those in sports where the stomach is relatively stable. Jostling seems to be a risk factor for abdominal distress; food eaten too close to such exercise time can often "talk back."

Walter, a 21-year-old triathlete and college student, eats according to his sport-of-the day. "When I bike, I enjoy a reasonable meal before the ride and munch on goodies during the workout, or even stop at the dairy for ice cream. When I run, I have to abstain from food for 3 hours before a workout, or else I get diarrhea. That's one reason I prefer biking to running."

Four Functions of Pre-Event Nourishment

Your pre-event/pre-exercise meal has four main functions:

1. To help prevent hypoglycemia (low blood sugar), with its symptoms of light-headedness, needless fatigue, blurred vision, and indecisiveness—all of which can interfere with top performance.
2. To help settle your stomach, absorb some of the gastric juices, and abate hunger feelings.
3. To fuel your muscles, particularly with food eaten far enough in advance to be digested and stored as glycogen.
4. To pacify your mind with the knowledge that your body is well-fueled.

To determine the right pretraining or precompetition meal for your body, experiment with the following 10 guidelines. You may find your preferences vary with type of exercise, level of intensity, and time of day.

1. Every day, eat high-carbohydrate meals to fuel and refuel your muscles so they'll be ready for action. Food eaten within an hour before exercise primarily keeps you from feeling hungry; it doesn't significantly replenish muscle glycogen stores.

2. Choose high-starch, low-fat foods—bread, English muffins, bagels, crackers, pasta, and so on—because these tend to digest easily, settle comfortably, and maintain a stable blood sugar. In comparison, high-fat proteins—cheese, steak, hamburgers, peanut butter—take longer to empty from the stomach because fat delays gastric emptying. Cheeseburgers with french fries, large ice cream cones, and pan-

cakes glistening with butter have been known to contribute to sluggishness.

Small servings of *low-fat* protein, however, can settle well. One 16-year-old gymnast likes having a scrambled egg for her precompetition breakfast; her brother, also a gymnast, prefers a small slice of cheese pizza. Here are some other appropriate choices:

- 2 or 3 thin slices of turkey or chicken (in a sandwich)
- 1 or 2 slices of lite cheese (in pita bread)
- A spoonful of low-fat cottage cheese (with canned peaches or pineapple)
- 1 or 2 poached eggs (on toast)
- 1 glass of skim milk (with cereal and banana)

3.   Avoid sugary foods, such as soft drinks, jelly beans, maple syrup, or even lots of fruit juice, within an hour before hard exercise. The sugar may give you a short-lived "sugar boost," but you are at risk of slumping into a "sugar low" once you start your workout. This hypoglycemia (low blood sugar) leaves you feeling light-headed and needlessly fatigued. (See chapter 4 for more information about sugar fixes before exercise.)

If you simply must have a little bit of something sweet, eat it within 5 to 10 minutes of exercise. This short time span is too brief for the body to secrete excess insulin, the hormone that causes low blood sugar. Because the body stops secreting insulin when you start to exercise, you should be able to handle this sugar fix safely *if* the food settles comfortably.

4.   Allow adequate time for food to digest. Remember that high-calorie meals take longer to leave the stomach than lighter snacks. The general "rule of thumb" is to allow

- 3 to 4 hours for a large meal to digest,
- 2 to 3 hours for a smaller meal,
- 1 to 2 hours for a blended or liquid meal, and
- less than an hour for a small snack, according to your own tolerance.

If you're going to participate in a 10:00 road race, you might want to eat only a light 200- to 400-calorie breakfast, such as a small bowl of cereal with low-fat milk at about 7:00 or 8:00. A hefty 700- to 800-calorie pancake breakfast might weigh you down. For a noon event, a hefty pancake breakfast at 8:00 could be adequately digested.

5.   Allow more digestion time before intense exercise than before low-level activity. Charley, a 42-year-old runner and physician, always allows 4 hours' digestion time prior to an intense track workout, but

he commonly munches on a bagel 10 minutes before a low-level training run. "If I have any food in my stomach before an all-out effort, I feel nauseous. Before an easy training run, however, I can eat almost anything with no stomach problems whatsoever."

Your muscles require more blood during intense exercise than when at rest so your stomach may get only 20 percent of its normal blood flow during a hard workout. This slows the digestive process. Any food in the stomach jostles along for the ride and may feel uncomfortable or be regurgitated.

During exercise of moderate intensity, blood flow to the stomach is 60 to 70 percent of normal, and you can still digest food. The snacks that recreational skiers, cyclists, and even ultra-runners eat before and during exercise do get digested and contribute to lasting energy during long-term, moderate-intensity events. On the adjacent page are some ideas to help you plan your pre-event mealtimes.

6. Liquid foods leave the stomach faster than solid foods. You might want to experiment with liquefied meals to see whether they offer you any advantage (see "Sample Liquid Meals," which follows). In one research study, a 450-calorie meal of steak, peas, and buttered bread remained in the stomach for 6 hours. A liquefied version of the same meal emptied from the stomach 2 hours earlier (Brouns, Saris, & Rehrer, 1987).

Before converting to liquid meals before events, keep in mind that some athletes report that too much liquid "sloshes" in the stomach and contributes to a nauseous feeling. Always experiment with any new food *during training* to see whether it offers you any advantage.

Sample Liquid Meals

Some athletes prefer liquid meals before games because they empty from the stomach more quickly than solid foods.

Cereal shake: 450 calories; 60% carbohydrate, 20% protein, 20% fat

Blend: 2 cups low-fat milk
1 cup favorite cereal
Small banana
4 ice cubes

Optional: 1/4 teaspoon vanilla, dash of cinnamon, 1 teaspoon sweetener.

Fruit shake: 470 calories; 75% carbohydrate, 15% protein, 10% fat

Blend: 1 cup vanilla yogurt
4–6 halves peaches, canned or fresh
4 graham cracker squares

Optional: Dash of nutmeg.

Timing Meals Before Events

Time: 8 a.m. event, such as a road race or swim meet

Meals: The night before, eat a high-carbohydrate dinner. Drink extra water. The morning of the event, about 6:00 or 6:30, have a light meal (depending on your tolerance), such as 2 slices of toast, tea or coffee if you like, and extra water. Eat familiar foods. If you want a bigger meal, you might want to get up to eat by 5:00 or 6:00.

Time: 10 a.m. event, such as a bike race or soccer game

Meals: The night before, eat a high-carbohydrate meal and drink extra water. The morning of the event, eat a familiar breakfast by 7:00, to allow 3 hours for the food to digest. This meal will prevent the fatigue that results from low blood sugar. If your body cannot handle any breakfast, eat a late snack before going to bed the night before. This will help boost liver glycogen stores and prevent low blood sugar the next morning.

Time: 2 p.m. event, such as a football or lacrosse game

Meals: An afternoon game allows time for you to have either a big, high-carbohydrate breakfast and a light lunch, or a substantial brunch by 10:00, allowing 4 hours for digestion time. As always, eat a high-carbohydrate dinner the night before, and drink extra fluids the day before and up to noontime.

Time: 8 p.m. event, such as a basketball game

Meals: A hefty, high-carbohydrate breakfast and lunch will be thoroughly digested by evening. Plan for dinner, as tolerated, by 5:00 or have a lighter meal between 6:00 and 7:00. Drink extra fluids all day.

Time: All-day event, such as a non-competitive 100-mile ride, triathlon training, or a long, hard hike

Meals: The day before, cut back on your exercise—take a rest day to allow your muscles the chance to replace depleted glycogen stores. Eat carbohydrate-rich meals at breakfast, lunch, and dinner. Drink extra fluids. The day of the event, eat breakfast depending on your tolerance—whatever you normally have before exercising.

Throughout the day, plan to snack every 1-1/2 to 2 hours on wholesome carbohydrates to maintain a normal blood sugar. At lunchtime, eat a low-fat meal. Drink fluids before you get thirsty; you should need to urinate at least 2 or 3 times throughout the day.

7.   If you know that you'll be jittery and unable to tolerate any food before an event, make a special effort to eat well the day before. Have an extra-large bedtime snack in lieu of breakfast. Some athletes can comfortably eat before they exercise, but others prefer to abstain. Both sorts perform well, and both have simply learned what works best for their bodies.

8.   If you have a "magic food," be sure to pack it along with you when traveling to an event—even if it's a standard item such as bananas—just so you will be certain to have it on hand.

Even if you have no favorite foods, you still might want to pack something. If you should encounter delays, like being stuck in traffic or stranded at an airport, you'd still be able to eat adequately. Emergency foods might include "durable" carbohydrates that don't easily crumble—for instance, fig bars, dried fruits, bread sticks, or bagels.

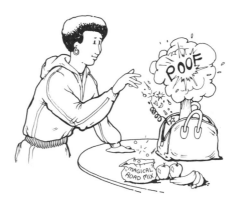

9.   Always eat familiar foods before a competition. Don't try anything new! Pete, a competitive skier, read about a new sports drink that was supposed to be the greatest formula available for nourishment before a race. He tried some before a championship event. What a mistake! The liquid gave him a sour stomach; and he felt nauseous and performed poorly. He would have been far better off staying with his tried-and-true oatmeal.

Like many athletes, Pete learned the hard way that he should experiment with new foods only during training. New foods always carry the risk of settling poorly, necessitating "pit stops," or causing intestinal discomfort, "acid stomach," heartburn, or cramps. Schedule a few workouts of intensity similar to and at the same time of day as an upcoming competition, and experiment with different foods to determine which (and how much) will be best on race day. *Never* try anything new before a competition, unless you want to risk impairing your performance.

10. Drink plenty of fluids. You're unlikely to starve to death during an event, but you might dehydrate.

- Drink an extra four to eight glasses of fluid the day before, so that you overhydrate. You should have to urinate frequently.
- Drink at least two or three large glasses of water up to 2 hours before the event.
- Drink another one or two glasses 5 to 10 minutes before the start. For more information about fluids, see chapter 10.

Feeding Both Muscles and Mind

For some athletes, food eaten before exercise has more psychological than physiological power. For example, Tim, a cyclist, just *has* to eat cereal before any bike race. No other breakfast is adequate. He carries his cereal and fruit with him whenever he travels to a race, and feels handicapped unless his appetite is satisfied with muesli topped with a well-ripened banana.

Tim swears that his breakfast contributes not only to strong, successful performances but also to high-quality training and overall well-being. He's confident that the carbohydrates, potassium, calcium, and other nutrients help him win. Undoubtedly they do—if not physiologically, at least psychologically!

Without a doubt, your mind can very powerfully convert any ordinary food into energy-enhancing fuel. Although this attachment to a ''special'' food can be helpful, it can also be harmful if the food is unavailable. You may feel handicapped without your magic morsel.

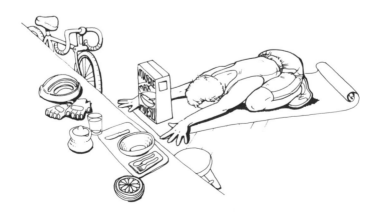

For example, one of my clients, a runner, felt "crippled" when competing in Italy because he couldn't find bran muffins, his favorite food before events.

Carbo-Loading for Endurance Exercise

Eating a high-carbohydrate diet for 1 day can adequately fuel your muscles with glycogen for a short event that lasts less than 90 non-stop minutes. If you're preparing for an endurance event that lasts more than 90 grueling minutes—a competitive marathon, triathlon, cross-country ski race, or long distance bike race—you'll want to eat carbohydrate-rich foods for 2 to 3 days beforehand to supersaturate your muscles with glycogen. During competition you'll be draining yourself of all you've got stored, so every little bit of glycogen will be important.

Most athletes prefer to eat their standard training diet before a marathon. Their biggest change is to

- cut back on exercise,
- rest the muscles, and
- allow the muscles to supersaturate with carbohydrates.

If you make major changes, such as trying to carbo-load on fruits that you rarely eat, you may discover to your disappointment that drastic dietary changes result in gastrointestinal distress.

Here is my 8-step carbohydrate-loading plan for all endurance athletes:

1. *Carbo-load every day.* That is, every training day you should eat a diet that's high in carbohydrates and low in fats and offers a moderate amount of protein. This 60 to 70 percent carbohydrate intake (equivalent to about 300 to 400 grams of carbohydrate for an average-size woman, and 500 to 600 grams for an average-size man) prevents chronic glycogen depletion and allows you to train and compete at your best. Too many endurance athletes suffer from chronic glycogen depletion because they carbo-load only a few days prior to a competition. By counting grams of carbohydrates, as suggested in chapter 7, you'll be able to know if your sports diet hits this target.

2. *Eat primarily tried-and-true carbohydrates beginning 3 days before competition.* They will supersaturate your muscles with glycogen and help protect you from "hitting the wall." Reduce your exercise time and rest your muscles, allowing them the opportunity to fuel up with these carbohydrates (refer to the following diet exercise guide).

Diet and Exercise Guide for Endurance Athletes

Before an endurance event of more than 90 minutes of hard effort, you can superfuel your muscles by following this plan:

Number of days before race	Exercise time frame	Training diet: % carbohydrates
6	90 min	60%
5	40 min	60%
4	40 min	60%
3	20 min	70%
2	20 min	70%
1	Rest day	70%
Race	Go for it!	Meal before event, depending on your tolerance

Caution: When you reduce your exercise, you'll need fewer calories. You may be eating less food but needing a higher percentage of carbohydrates. You'll know you've properly loaded if you've gained 2 to 4 pounds (water weight). With each ounce of stored glycogen, you store 3 ounces of water. This water becomes available during exercise and reduces dehydration.

Note. Based on information from "Effect of Exercise-Diet Manipulation on Muscle Glycogen Storage and Its Subsequent Utilization During Performance," by W. Sherman, et al., 1981, *International Journal of Sports Medicine,* **2**, pp. 114-118. Adapted by permission.

3. *Don't fat-load.* Have toast with jam rather than butter, pancakes moist with maple syrup rather than slick with margarine, pasta with tomato sauce rather than with oil and cheese (as in fettucini alfredo), pizza with extra crust rather than extra cheese.

Your goal is to get about 65 to 70 percent of your calories from carbohydrates. To do that, you'll have to trade in most of the fat calories for more carbohydrates—for example, have two baked potatoes (300 calories) rather than one potato with two pats of butter and a dollop of sour cream (300 calories). You may have to eat a lot of food to get enough calories. For example, a 1-pound box of spaghetti cooks into a mountain of pasta but is only 1,600 calories. That's a reasonable calorie goal for a hefty premarathon meal, but it may be more volume than you want.

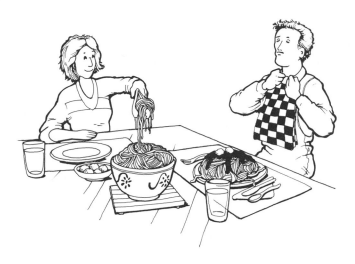

4.   *Choose wholesome, fiber-rich carbohydrates*. These promote regular bowel movements and keep your system "running smoothly." Bran muffins, whole wheat bread, bran cereal, fruits, and vegetables are some good choices. If you eat too much white bread, pasta, rice, and other refined products, you're likely to get constipated, particularly if you're doing less training. See the section on fiber in chapter 2 for more information.

If you're fiber-sensitive and worried about diarrhea, you should avoid fiber-rich foods before an event.

5.   *Plan meal times carefully*. On the day before the event, you might want to eat your biggest meal at lunchtime so that the food will have plenty of time to digest and pass through your system. Later, enjoy a normal-size dinner and a bedtime snack. One runner discovered with dismay that an exceptionally hefty dinner she ate the night before a marathon was still sitting heavily in her system come marathon morning.

6.   *Drink extra fluids to hydrate your body*. This reduces your risk of becoming dehydrated.

- Drink four to eight extra glasses of water and juices daily, on the day or two before the event. You should have to urinate frequently.
- Limit dehydrating fluids such as beer, wine, and other alcoholic beverages and those containing caffeine.

- On race morning, drink at least three glasses of water up to 2 hours before the event, and one or two glasses 5 to 10 minutes before race time. (For more information on fluids, see chapter 10.)

7. *On the morning of the event, eat a light breakfast* (according to your tolerance) to prevent hunger and help maintain a normal blood sugar level. As part of your training, you should have "practiced" eating before races to learn which foods in what amount work best for you.

8. *Be sensible!* Don't carbo-load on only fruit or you're likely to get diarrhea. Don't carbo-load on only refined white bread products or you're likely to become constipated. Don't carbo-load on beer or you'll get dehydrated. Don't do too much last-minute training or you'll fatigue your muscles.

Caffeine: A Stimulating Topic

Will caffeine help you perform better? Some folks say yes, while others disagree.

Before he races, Pat, a 27-year-old swimmer, always drinks a cup of coffee. "Maybe the effect is psychological, but I think that caffeine enhances my performance. My muscles seem to work more easily."

Jean, a soccer player, avoids the stuff. "A cup of coffee before a game would put me over the edge. I'm already jittery, and a caffeine-jag is the last thing I need!"

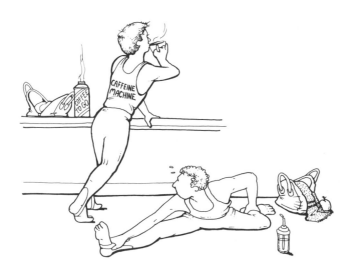

Henry, a runner, prefers his coffee after exercise. "Drinking coffee on an empty stomach makes me nauseous. I prefer my brew after I run, as I relax with a nice meal and the morning paper."

For some folks, coffee is a priceless "perk-me-up" before exercise. For others, it's a worthless beverage that simply makes them jittery and discomforted by coffee stomach. Researchers have suggested that caffeine can significantly enhance an athlete's endurance. In one study (Costill, 1978), runners who had the caffeine equivalent of 2 cups of coffee—330 mg caffeine—1 hour prior to exhaustive running ran 15 minutes longer than when they exercised to exhaustion without caffeine.

Based on that study, you might conclude that caffeine offers an advantage for endurance athletes. Supposedly, caffeine before exercise stimulates the release of fat into the blood, and the muscles theoretically burn this abundant fuel rather than the limited muscle-glycogen stores. Endurance athletes should be able to exercise longer before glycogen depletion causes them to hit the wall.

Since this and other reports on caffeine's energy-enhancing effect, the topic of caffeine and athletic performance has become controversial among exercise physiologists and athletes alike. Some claim caffeine has a significant energy-enhancing effect; other researchers are doubtful.

In the original studies, caffeine was examined alone—not in context of the athlete's diet and training program. More recently, investigators found no energy advantages from caffeine prior to exercise when the subjects (well-trained runners) had eaten carbohydrate-rich diets and tapered their training, as one might do prior to a marathon; these results suggest that carbo-loading, more than caffeine, is the bigger ergogenic aid for endurance athletes (Weir, 1987). Regardless, caffeine is a drug banned by the U.S. Olympic Committee.

Caffeine as a Drug

Although small doses of caffeine, as in a morning cup of coffee, are permissible, the International Olympic Committee has put large doses of caffeine on the banned list. Olympians with more than 12 micrograms of caffeine per milliliter of urine can be disqualified from competition. To get this level, one would have to deliberately consume in 2 or 3 hours the equivalent of one of the following:

- 8 coffees
- 16 colas
- 24 Anacin
- 4 Vivarin

This is clearly an abnormally high amount.

Caffeine's potential energy-enhancing effect is related not only to the pre-event meal, but also to the individual's tolerance to caffeine. Some people are very caffeine sensitive—a small cup of coffee wires them for hours!

Others feel dehydrated due to caffeine's diuretic effect. One basketball player I counseled avoided coffee before games; otherwise, he'd be running too often to the bathroom. "Coffee stomach" is another common complaint among people who exercise with nothing in their stomach but a mugful of brew. They feel lousy and quickly learn never to do that again!

Too much caffeine can reduce performance. Just because a little bit may be good, a lot may not be better! I often talk with athletes who've learned through trial and error that the second mugful did them in with the caffeine jitters. Table 8.1 lists the caffeine amounts in some common perk-me-ups.

Table 8.1 Caffeine in Beverages

Beverage	Amount	Caffeine (mg)
Brewed coffee	8 oz	100–150
Instant coffee	8 oz	85–100
Decaffeinated coffee	8 oz	5
Tea	8 oz	60–75
Cocoa	8 oz	5–40
Cola	12 oz	40–60

Note. From T. Leonard, R. Watson, and M. Mohs. "The Effects of Caffeine on Various Body Systems: A Review." Copyright The American Association. Reprinted by permission from *Journal of the American Dietetic Association,* **87**: 1048, 1987.

Caffeine Comfort

One reason for drinking caffeinated beverages before exercise may be caffeine's ability to make exercise seem easier, perhaps by stimulating the nervous system. In one study, subjects "pedalled" as hard as they could for 2 hours on special bicycles that recorded the amount of energy they expended. They worked 7 percent harder after taking caffeine than when they cycled without it, despite perceiving the efforts as equal (Ivy, 1979).

I've heard many athletes agree a small cup of coffee makes the effort seem easier. I personally savor 1 teaspoon of coffee diluted into a large mug of water for my preexercise beverage of choice. Be it physiological or psychological, this tiny potion seems to help me run better!

However, many folks drink a warm mug of coffee not for an energy boost, but because it cleans them out and promotes regular bowel movements. Warm liquids have a laxative effect. This may be the best reason of all for including this brew in your sports diet!

For more information on caffeine as a part of your daily diet, see chapter 2.

Transit Problems: Constipation and Diarrhea

Most athletes go to great extremes to promote bowel regularity and prevent discomfort or pit stops during exercise. They religiously eat fiber-rich foods to prevent constipation, drink warm liquids in the morning to encourage regular bowel movements, eat plenty of fresh fruits and vegetables, and drink more than enough fluids. Other athletes have the opposite problem—rapid transit. Diarrhea can be caused by food intolerances or training too much or too fast. If you have persistent problems with diarrhea, intestinal distress, and gastrointestinal (GI) cramping, you should consult a registered dietitian or sports nutritionist. Don't make radical long-term dietary changes without the concurrence of someone knowledgeable about nutrition. Some folks have trouble with fruit, wheat, or milk. Athletes who can't tolerate milk, for example, need alternative, nondairy sources for the calcium, riboflavin, and other nutrients in milk. A dietitian can help them choose substitutes without sacrificing nutrition.

One race-walker worked like a detective to determine the cause of her gastric distress. She was bothered by constant intestinal gas and bloating. She tried all of these strategies:

- Eliminating suspected problem foods to see if the problem went away; reintroducing them to see if it returned
- Allowing more time between eating and exercise
- Limiting broccoli, onions, corn, kidney beans, and other possible gas-forming foods
- Avoiding coffee and anything she could think of that might be a culprit

Nothing made any difference. She charted every food and fluid that she ate and drank, as well when she exercised and had GI problems, to try to determine a pattern.

The culprit turned out to be sugar-free chewing gum. It contains sorbitol, a type of sugar that can cause GI problems if taken in excess. This lady simply chewed too much gum—20 sticks a day! When she eliminated gum, her GI problems disappeared. What a simple solution to a perplexing problem.

Inappropriate training can also contribute to gastrointestinal problems. Peter, a jogger, was plagued with diarrhea when he started to increase his training mileage. I recommended that he cut back to his baseline mileage for a week, then gradually add on 1 to 2 miles per week, rather than 8 to 10. I also advised him to talk with a sports doctor to determine whether he had a medical problem. For Peter, the solution was training-related. He was trying to run too much, too fast. In most cases, well-trained athletes whose bodies have adapted to the stress of intense exercise have fewer GI problems than novices.

CHAPTER 9

Nutrition After Exercise: Recovery Foods

Billy, a 47-year-old runner, noticed that he wasn't recovering from the Boston Marathon as quickly as his peers; he wondered if a poor diet could make a difference.

Preparing for Boston, I ate a blue ribbon diet. I chose bran muffins instead of donuts, apples instead of Twinkies, spaghetti rather than burgers and fries. I really wanted to run well, and I ran my best time ever—2:32. Afterwards, I rewarded myself with chips, beer, steak, french fries, and ice cream. I felt tired and abnormally achy for more than a week. If I'd eaten better, would I have recovered faster?

Other competitive athletes have expressed similar concerns: Football players want to know what they should eat after morning practice to prepare for the afternoon session; body builders wonder if they should eat extra protein after workouts to repair muscles; tennis champs seek out foods that will prepare them for the next day's match.

What you eat after a hard workout or competition *can* affect your recovery. For the serious athlete, foods eaten after exercise require the same careful selections as the meal before exercising. By wisely choosing your foods and fluids, you'll recover more quickly for the next workout. It matters what you eat.

An optimal recovery diet is most important for athletes who do two or more workouts per day: football players at training camp who practice morning and afternoon, competitive swimmers who compete in multiple events per day, triathletes who train twice per day, aerobics instructors who teach several classes per day. In order to recover and refuel for the next bout, they should pay particular attention to what they eat after the first session.

This chapter outlines the most important considerations for optimal recovery from either exhaustive daily training, one hard competition, or multiple events in the same day or weekend. For more information, refer to the chapters on carbohydrate, fluids, and protein.

Recovery Fluids

After a hard workout, one of your priorities should be to replace the fluids you lost by sweating. The best choices for replacing these sweat losses include one or more of the following:

- Juices, which supply water, carbohydrates, and electrolytes
- Water, which tends to be a conventional and well-tolerated fluid
- Watery foods such as watermelon, grapes, and soups, which supply fluid, carbohydrates, vitamins, and minerals (electrolytes)
- High-carbohydrate sports drinks or soft drinks, which supply fluids and carbohydrates (but minimal, if any vitamins or minerals)

To determine how much water you lose during a strenuous event, weigh yourself before and after a hard training workout. You're goal is to lose no more than 2 percent of your body weight (that is, 3 pounds for a 150 pound person). One football player was shocked to discover that, on a relatively cool day, he'd lost 8 pounds during the morning football practice—5 percent of his body weight and the equivalent of a gallon of sweat! (One pound of sweat loss represents 2 cups of fluid.)

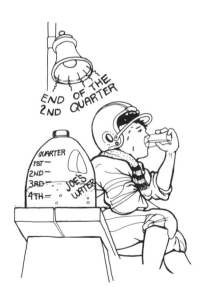

He became aware of the importance of drinking more water than he might have otherwise. He started to bring a water jug to practice so that he wouldn't feel guilty for taking more than his share from the limited water bucket on the playing field! He made sure that he drank that whole gallon—plus more on very hot days—between the morning and afternoon practices. He took steps to prevent dehydration to help him recovery easily.

If you become dehydrated during an unusually long and strenuous bout of exercise, you should drink frequently for the next day or two. Your body may need 24 to 48 hours to replace the sweat losses. You'll know that you're adequately rehydrated when your urine is clear and you have to urinate frequently. Dark-colored urine is still concentrated with metabolic wastes.

Recovery Carbohydrates

You should consume carbohydrate-rich foods and beverages within 1 to 4 hours after your workout (see Figure 9.1). The target intake is 0.5 grams of carbohydrates per pound of body weight within the first 2 hours. Repeat this amount 2 hours later.

Let's assume that you weigh 150 pounds:

150 lb x 0.5 g carbohydrates/lb = 75 g carbohydrates

Thus, you need about 75 grams of carbohydrate within the first 2 hours. One gram of carbohydrate contains 4 calories, so this converts to 300 calories. Two hours later, you should eat another 300 calories of high-carbohydrate foods. You can get at least 300 carbohydrate calories in

- 1 cup of orange juice and a bagel
- 2 cups of cranberry juice
- 1 12-ounce can of soft drink (not diet) and an 8-ounce fruit yogurt
- 1 bowl of cereal with a banana

High-carbohydrate sports drinks, such as Gatorade and Exceed High Carbohydrate, can also refuel your muscles. But be aware that these types of fluids often lack the vitamins and minerals found in wholesome foods.

Most fitness enthusiasts recover at their own pace because they don't deplete their glycogen stores in their typical 20-to-30-minute workout. Hard-core endurance athletes, on the other hand, should monitor their diets carefully to ensure proper refueling.

One cyclist knew that she should eat carbohydrates after racing, but she was tired of pasta; she wanted meat. Like many endurance athletes, she'd eaten primarily carbs for the 3 days prior to her event

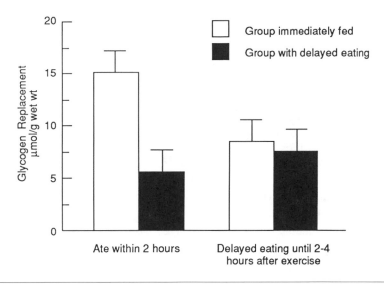

Figure 9.1. *Note:* From "Muscle Glycogen Synthesis After Exercise and Effect of Time Carbohydrate Ingestion" by J. Ivy, et al., 1988, *Journal of Applied Physiology,* **64**, p. 1480-1485. Copyright 1988 by the American Physiological Society. Adapted by permission.

and now wanted something else. She satisfied this craving and properly refueled her muscles by eating a hamburger supplemented with lots of carbohydrates: a thick kaiser roll, minestrone soup with crackers, lemonade, and fruit yogurt. The hamburger became an accompaniment to the other carbohydrate-rich choices, and she ended up with a high-carbohydrate diet after all.

Although *extra* protein is unnecessary after exercise, you do need the RDA for protein. In some cases, carbohydrate-conscious athletes shun protein, forgetting that adequate amounts are essential for a well-balanced diet that sustains overall good health. They should include some protein to balance out their diet.

Recovery Electrolytes

Along with the water in sweat, you do lose some minerals (electrolytes), such as sodium and potassium, that help your body function normally. You can easily replace these losses with the foods and fluids you consume after the event. Based on the assumption that the harder you exercise, the hungrier you'll get and the more you'll eat, you'll consume more than enough electrolytes from food. You won't need salt tablets or special supplements. For example, Pete guzzled a whole quart of orange juice after his 2:32 marathon. This replaced 3 times the potassium he might have lost. A third of a quart, which contains 600 milligrams of potassium, would have done the job! He also munched on a bag of pretzels and more than replaced sodium losses.

Potassium

Although potassium-rich orange juice is a particularly good choice for a recovery fluid, for many athletes it is too acidic and settles uncomfortably. Alternatives include almost any natural juices, such as pineapple juice or apricot nectar—they all offer some potassium. Another alternative is to drink plain water for fluid and eat a banana for potassium. See Table 9.1 for potassium-rich recovery foods.

Table 9.1   Potassium in Some Popular Recovery Foods

During 2 to 3 hours of hard exercise, you might lose 300 to 800 milligrams of potassium at about 80 to 100 milligrams potassium per pound of sweat. The following chart rank-orders some fluids and foods for potassium content. In general, natural foods are preferable to commercial products. See Tables 1.3, 1.4, and 2.7 for a more complete potassium list.

Recovery foods	Potassium (mg)
Potato, 3″	750
Yogurt, 1 c	500
Banana, med	500
Orange juice, 1 c	420
Pineapple juice, 1 c	360
Raisins, 1/4 c	300
Beer, 12 oz	90
Exceed fluid replacer, 1 c	25
Gatorade, 1 c	24
Coke, 12 oz	5

Note. Nutrient data from *Bowes and Church's Food Values of Portions Commonly Used* (14th ed.) by J. Pennington and H. Church, 1985, Philadelphia: Lippincott. Adapted by permission.

If you're tempted to replace potassium losses with commercially prepared fluid replacement beverages, remember that most of these special sports drinks are potassium-poor. Compare these two to orange juice, which has 420 milligrams of potassium:

- 8 ounces of Gatorade has only 24 milligrams of potassium
- 8 ounces of Exceed has only 45 milligrams of potassium

Commercial fluid replacement drinks are designed to be taken during intense exercise. They are very dilute, which helps them to empty faster from the stomach. They are not the best recovery foods in terms of electrolyte content, carbohydrates, and overall nutritional value.

Sodium

Another electrolyte that you lose when you sweat is sodium (a part of salt). Although you lose a little sodium under ordinary exercise conditions, you do not come close to depleting your body's stores. For the average fitness participant, replacing salt losses either after or during exercise is of no major concern.

In most cases, the typical American diet more than adequately replaces sodium losses. Popular recovery foods such as yogurt, muffins, pizza, and spaghetti have more sodium than you may realize! If you need extra salt, you'll crave it. Sprinkle a little on your food, or choose some salty items such as pretzels, crackers, or soup.

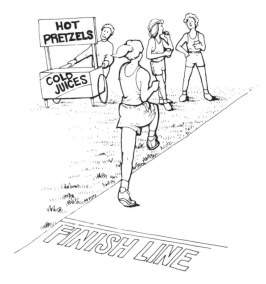

In extreme circumstances, such as an ultra-endurance event that lasts for hours in the heat, you have a higher risk of becoming sodium depleted. To prevent this, be sure to consume salted fluids or foods during the event (see Table 9.2).

Rest

The day after his marathon, Dave felt compelled to hop back on his feet and start training for the next event 2 months away. "I feel guilty

Table 9.2 Sodium in Some Popular Recovery Foods

During 2 to 3 hours of hard exercise, you might lose 1,800 to 5,600 milligrams of sodium at about 400 to 700 milligrams sodium per pound of sweat. The more you're adapted to exercising in the heat, the less sodium you'll lose. If you need salt, you'll crave it.

Recovery Foods	Sodium (mg)
Pizza, 1/2 med	1,400
Vegetable soup, 1/2 can	1,250
Spaghetti sauce, 2/3 c	1,000
Chow mein, 1 c	1,000
Salt, 1 small packet	500
Cheese, 1 oz American	400
Saltines, 6	300
Pretzels, 6 (3-ring)	300
Gatorade, 1 c	130
Beer, 12 oz	25
Coke, 12 oz	25
Orange juice, 8 oz	5

if I don't run every day. I'm afraid I'll become weak, fat, and lazy if I miss a day of training.''

Like many compulsive exercisers, Dave allowed no recovery time in his exercise program. He neglected the important physiological fact that rest is essential for top performances. I told him that rest would enhance his recovery process as well as his future performances.

Time is necessary for the recovery process. To completely replace depleted glycogen stores, the muscles need about 2 rest days with no exercise and a high-carbohydrate diet. There's no way Dave could have done quality training with his battered muscles.

Dave admitted that he was being compulsive and not wise. I suggested that, rather than attempt a training run on the day after a major event, he try an alternative form of exercise that would limber up his tight muscles but not pound his joints. He took a gentle bike ride to the swimming pool and slowly swam laps for 15 minutes, easing his guilty conscience and loosening his muscles. Dave's muscles were sorer by the second day after the marathon, but this achiness is normal. Most athletes experience worse soreness on the second day after strenuous exercise. If the pain persists, they should consult a sports medicine specialist for some professional help. And, of course, they should keep eating a variety of wholesome foods with all the vitamins, minerals, and protein needed to enhance the healing process.

CHAPTER 10

Fluid Facts for Thirsty Athletes

The same athletes who earn an A+ for eating wisely often flunk hydration. One runner, for example, routinely neglected to drink adequate fluids during training or before competitions. He became needlessly fatigued, trained poorly, and did not perform at his best. This oversight cost him his desired personal record at several events. When he began drinking additional fluids on a daily basis, he felt more enthusiastic and noticed that he had greater energy and faster times.

Fluids and You

Drinking adequate fluid is essential for top athletic performance because body fluids have important jobs:

- Fluid in *blood* transports glucose to working muscles and carries away metabolic by-products.
- Fluid in *urine* eliminates metabolic waste products.
- Fluid in *sweat* dissipates heat through the skin.

If you drink too little fluid, or lose too much through profuse sweating, you inhibit your body's ability to accomplish these tasks, which prevents you from exercising at your maximum potential.

Under extreme conditions, dehydrated athletes suffer severe medical complications. Some individuals have died because misinformed coaches told them never to drink before or during training. Water was once thought to cause stomach cramping, but now we know that you should drink as much water as you comfortably can before, during, and after exercise.

To help dispel confusion about fluids and dehydration, here are the answers to questions commonly asked by thirsty athletes.

Sweating it Out

Q. *I sweat buckets! After a workout, I'm dripping wet and leave puddles on the floor. Is this healthy?*

A. Sweating is good for you! It's the body's way of dissipating heat and maintaining constant internal temperature (98.6 °F). During hard exercise, you may generate 20 times more heat than when you're at rest. You dissipate this heat by sweating. As the sweat evaporates, it cools the skin; this in turn cools the blood, and that cools the inner body. If you did not sweat, you could conceivably "cook" yourself to death. A body temperature higher than 106 °F damages the cells. At 107.6 °F, cell protein coagulates (as do egg whites when they cook), and the cell dies. This is one serious reason why you shouldn't push yourself beyond your limits in very hot weather.

An athlete loses about 2 cups (1 pound) of sweat for every 300 calories of heat she or he dissipates. Men tend to sweat more than women of equal body size. Plus, men tend to lose more total sweat than women because they generally weigh more and therefore burn off more calories at the same level of exertion.

Women tend to sweat more efficiently than men. Women sweat small droplets of water that evaporate easily. Men tend to sweat larger drops, which can drip off the skin rather than evaporate, resulting in a lessened cooling effect.

Replacing Losses

Q. *How do I know whether I'm drinking enough fluids to replace the sweat?*

A. The simplest way to tell if you're adequately replacing sweat losses is to check the color and quantity of your urine. If your urine is very dark and scanty, it is concentrated with metabolic wastes, and you need to drink more fluids. When your urine is a clear color, your body has returned to its normal water balance. Your urine may be dark if you're taking vitamin supplements; in that case, volume is a better indicator than color.

Another way to monitor sweat loss is to weigh yourself before and after you exercise. For every pound you lose, you should drink 2 cups of fluid. In hot weather, athletes may easily sweat off 5 to 8 pounds. The weight drop is water loss, not fat loss.

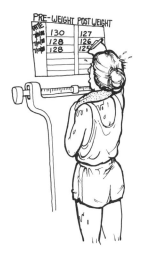

In addition to monitoring urine and weight loss, you should also pay attention to how you feel. If you are chronically fatigued, headachy, or needlessly lifeless, then you may be chronically dehydrated. This is most likely to happen during long hot spells in the summertime.

During a very hot week of preseason training, one football player drank like a camel but still couldn't get into water balance. He didn't urinate all day! He dragged through double training sessions and wilted with exhaustion after practice. He sweat so much that he wasn't adequately replacing the fluid loss even overnight; his morning urine was dark and scanty. By the third day into the heat wave, the coach recognized these symptoms of chronic dehydration in many of the players and wisely curtailed practices.

Q. *Does my thirst tell me if I've had enough to drink?*

A. No. You may not feel thirsty, yet you may need more fluids. Your safest bet is to judge by the color and quantity of your urine.

The sensation of thirst is triggered by an abnormally high concentration of sodium (a part of salt) in the blood. When you sweat, you lose significant amounts of water from your blood. The remaining blood becomes more concentrated and has an abnormally high sodium level. This triggers the thirst mechanism and increases your desire to drink. To quench your thirst, you have to replace the water losses and bring the blood back to its normal concentration.

Unfortunately for athletes, this thirst mechanism can be unreliable. To be on the safe side, always drink enough to quench your thirst, and then a little more.

Young children have a poorly developed thirst mechanism. At the end of a hot day, they often become very irritable, which may be partially due to dehydration. If you're going to spend the day with children at a place where fluids are not readily available, such as at the beach, bringing a cooler stocked with lemonade, juice, and water can increase everyone's enjoyment of the day!

Senior citizens also tend to be less sensitive to thirst sensations than younger adults. Research with active, healthy men aged 67 to 75 years old shows that they were less thirsty and voluntarily drank less water when water-deprived for 24 hours than similarly deprived men aged 20 to 31 years (Phillips, 1984). Senior citizens who participate in any sports should monitor their fluid intake.

Q. *How much should I drink before exercise?*

A. The exact amount you should drink depends on how large you are (for example, a slight wrestler would drink less than a hulky football player) and how much your stomach can comfortably handle. Although you'll have to learn your exact needs through trial and error, here are the general guidelines:

- Eliminate the risk of chronic dehydration. Quench your thirst, and then drink some more, especially if the weather is hot or if you've been training hard. You should have to urinate frequently throughout the day. Don't wait for the last-minute, "band-aid" approach to correct dehydration.
- Consume beverages, ideally water, up to 2 hours prior to a competitive event. Because the kidneys require about 60 to 90 minutes to process excess liquid, you'll have the chance to eliminate any excess before the competition. For example, if your event is at 10 a.m., drink 2 to 3 cups or more of fluids by 8 a.m.
- Drink 1 or 2 cups of water 5 to 15 minutes before your workout or competition. This fluid in your system will be ready to replace sweat losses.

Q. *How much should I drink during exercise?*

A. During any sporting event you should start drinking fluids early to prevent dehydration. What you consume at the start will invest in your finish, whether your event is a marathon, a soccer game, or a hike. In hot weather, drink as much as you can as often as you can. Ideally, this will be 8 to 10 ounces for every 15 or 20 minutes of strenuous exercise. Under extreme conditions, you might be sweating 3 times this amount, so that amount of fluid intake would still leave you with a deficit, but it can significantly reduce the drop in performance that accompanies dehydration.

Always drink before you're thirsty. By the time your brain signals thirst, you may have lost 1 percent of your body weight, which is the equivalent of 1.5 pounds (3 cups) of sweat for a 150-pound person. A 2-percent loss may reduce your work capacity by 10 to 15 percent of your maximum potential. That could be the difference between winning and losing.

Q. *Do I really need to drink eight glasses of water a day?*

A. Eight glasses of water might be adequate for a sedentary person, but it's probably too little for many athletes. A general rule of thumb is to consume a liter of water (about 1 quart) for every 1,000 calories you expend.

Rather than count glasses of fluid, you should drink liquids with each meal and monitor your urine output. If you're making frequent trips to the bathroom, you're probably drinking enough! In hot weather, drink a little more than you are thirsty for, to protect against chronic dehydration. You're unlikely to "drown yourself" by drinking too much fluid. If you drink more than your body needs, you'll pass the excess fluid through your system.

You don't have to drink water, per se, to meet your water requirements. Almost any nonalcoholic fluid, such as these, will do:

Seltzer	Lemonade
Juice	Soft drinks
Decaffeinated coffee or tea	Soups
Herbal tea	Low-fat milk

Even watery foods such as oranges and cucumbers contribute significant amounts of liquids (see below). Caffeine has a dehydrating effect; choose herbal tea, decaffeineated iced tea, or decaffeinated coffee for optimal hydration.

Watery Foods

Foods	% Water
Lettuce	95
Cucumber	95
Tomato	95
Orange	85
Banana	75
Chicken	60
Cheese	35
Cookie	5

If you get bored of drinking plain water, try seltzer. This sparkling alternative is calorie free, 100-percent pure, and filled with fun bubbles. Add a wedge of lime or a splash of juice for flavor. Any beverage that enhances fluid intake is a wise investment in top performance.

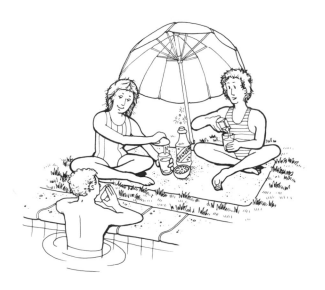

Fluid Choices

Q. *Does drinking cold water shock the system or cause stomach cramps?*

A. For the average, healthy athlete, drinking cold water does not shock the system or cause stomach cramps. In fact, during hot weather your best bet is to drink a cold fluid. It will not only cool you off faster, but it also will empty from your stomach faster than a warmer fluid. Research by exercise physiologist Dr. David Costill indicates that about one half of refrigerator-temperature (40 °F) water empties from the stomach in 20 minutes, as compared to only one fourth of warmer (90 °F) water in that length of time (Costill, 1974).

However, drinking cold water in the *winter* can be a poor choice. If you're skiing, hiking, or ice skating in cold weather, you might want to bring along a thermos filled with a warm soup or beverage to help you warm your body.

Q. *Is a soft drink a bad fluid replacement?*

A. Coke and Pepsi are among the more popular thirst quenchers for sports-active Americans, but they offer zero nutritional value except for 150 calories of refined sugar. This sugar does refuel the muscles with carbohydrates, but the natural sugars in juices also do the same trick. Juices also replace the potassium lost in sweat and offer vitamin C, a nutrient that promotes healing. Drinking soft drinks is like putting gas in the car but neglecting to put in spark plugs. Commercial sports drinks such as Gatorade, Max, or Exceed, also are sugar-ladened beverages that offer very little nutritional value (see Table 10.1).

Table 10.1   Thirst Quenchers

The best sports drinks offer not only adequate fluids and carbohydrates, but also vitamins and minerals. Soft drinks and commercial fluid replacers lack these and most other nutrients. Ounce for ounce, juices provide better quality nutrition.

Fluid, amount	Calories	Carbohydrates	C	B_2	A	Calcium
Cola, 8 oz	100	25	—	—	—	—
Gatorade, 8 oz	40	10	—	8	—	3
Orange juice, 8 oz	105	26	200	3	5	3

Note. Nutrient data from *Bowes and Church's Food Values of Portions Commonly Used* (14th ed.) by J. Pennington and H. Church, 1985, Philadelphia: Lippincott. Adapted by permission.

Rather than judging soft drinks as good or bad, I look at how many a person is consuming per day.

- A thirsty football player who enjoys a single can of cola can easily fit this 150 calories into his overall, wholesome, 5,000-plus calories per day.
- A petite gymnast who spends 450 of her 1,400-calories-per-day training diet on three soft drinks should reevaluate her choices. Obviously, moderation is the key word.

Drinking a sugar-free rather than a sugar-sweetened soft drink saves about 150 calories or the equivalent of 9 teaspoons of sugar. One or two diet sodas can add enjoyment to a reduction diet, but I advise against drinking liters of diet soft drinks every day; try mineral water or seltzer instead! Diet soft drinks have no positive nutritional content and may have negative side effects that we have yet to discover.

Sweet Satisfaction

Many nutrition-cautious athletes avoid artificial sweeteners. Nutra-sweet (aspartame) in particular has been controversial because some people report that it gives them headaches.

Most researchers believe that aspartame is harmless because it is made of two amino acids, aspartic acid and phenylalanine, that naturally occur in protein. Others suspect that phenylalanine may have adverse effects on certain people.

If sugar-free soft drinks are an enjoyable part of your diet, the safest advice is to drink them in moderation. One or two cans per day are unlikely to have any negative effects, but we don't yet know the long-term implications of ingesting large amounts of artificial sweeteners.

The following list compares the phenylalanine content of commonly eaten foods and beverages.

Item	Amount	Phenylalanine
Equal	1 pkt	35 mg
Diet soda	12 oz	180–200 mg
Skim milk	8 oz	400 mg
Tuna	3 oz	900 mg
Beef	4 oz	1,300 mg

Note. Nutrient data from *Bowes and Church's Food Values of Portions Commonly Used* (14th ed.) by J. Pennington and H. Church, 1985, Philadelphia: Lippincott. Adapted by permission.

Q. *I've heard that beer is a good sports drink because it's filled with carbohydrates, potassium, and B vitamins. Is this true?*

A. False! Beer is a *poor* sports drink for many reasons:

• *The alcohol in beer has a dehydrating effect.* If you drink beer after exercise, you'll take frequent trips to the bathroom and lose—rather than replace—valuable fluids. Drinking beer before an event increases your chances of dehydration during the event.

• *Beer is a poor source of carbohydrates.* Of the 150 calories in a 12-ounce can of beer, only 50 are from carbohydrates. The rest are from alcohol. Your muscles don't store alcohol calories as glycogen, so with beer you're more likely to get "loaded" than "carbo-loaded." Lite beer has even fewer carbohydrates (see Table 10.2).

• *Beer is a poor source of B vitamins.* You'd have to drink 11 cans of beer to get the RDA for riboflavin and a lot more to get other vita-

Table 10.2 Alcoholic Beverages

You can "get loaded" with alcohol, but you can't load your muscles with carbohydrates at the same time. The calories from beer, wine, and whiskey come mostly from the alcohol content. They are not converted into glycogen stores.

Beverage	Amount	Total calories	Carbohydrate-calories
Beer	12 oz	150	50
Lite beer	12 oz	100	24
Apricot brandy	1 cordial glass	65	25
80 proof whiskey	1.5 oz (jigger)	95	—
90 proof whiskey	1.5 oz (jigger)	110	—
Red wine	7 oz	150	20
White wine	7 oz	160	30
Dry vermouth	7 oz	210	10
Sweet vermouth	7 oz	330	100

Note. Nutrient data from *Bowes and Church's Food Values of Portions Commonly Used* (14th ed.) by J. Pennington and H. Church, 1985, Philadelphia: Lippincott. Adapted by permission.

mins in significant amounts. I always recommend that athletes get B vitamins from wholesome foods.

If you drink an occasional beer for social reasons, drink plenty of water also. If you're going to drink beer after an event, first quench your thirst with two or three large glasses of water. Then limit yourself to one or two beers.

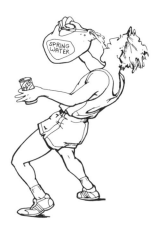

Q. *After a sweaty workout, I'm left with a thin layer of salt residue on my skin. Should I eat more salt to replace this loss?*

A. Generally not. Although you may think that you lose a significant amount of salt (more accurately, sodium, a part of salt) when you sweat, you far from deplete your body's supply. In research studies, athletes who lost about 6 percent of their body weight during a workout (the equivalent weight loss of 9 pounds for a 150-pound person) lost only 5 to 7 percent of their body's sodium supply. This is the equivalent of 3,000 to 4,800 milligrams of sodium. A teaspoon of salt contains 2,300 milligrams.

As I mentioned before, the concentration of in sodium in your blood actually increases during exercise because you lose proportionately more water than sodium. Your first need is to replace the fluid; you'll get adequate sodium in the food you eat.

Long-distance triathletes and other endurance athletes who exercise for more than 4 hours in extreme heat have a slight risk of developing medical problems from losing too much salt. If they replace extreme sweat losses with too much plain water, they may become metabolically imbalanced. They can prevent this by eating some salty foods or drinking sports drinks during the event. For us ordinary mortals, salt depletion is unlikely.

Sodium losses are easily replaced during your recovery meal after exercise. The average American diet contains 3 to 12 times more sodium than you need. Sodium occurs naturally in most food items, so you'll get plenty even if you do not add salt to your food. Fruits and juices (popular recovery foods) generally have a low sodium content, but yogurt, cheese, crackers, and pizza (equally popular choices) can do the job.

If you've been exercising strenuously in the heat for an extended period, such as a 100-mile bike ride or an all-day mountain climb with a heavy pack, you might crave salty foods. One cyclist commented that after hard summer training rides he seeks out pretzels, popcorn, and other salty snacks. "The salt tastes good to me—I tend to crave it."

Such cravings are your body's way of telling you that you need extra salt. You might want to sprinkle some on your recovery meal. The chances are good that after doing the amount of exercise needed to trigger this craving, you'll be very hungry and will consume more than enough sodium in the large helpings of food you'll devour.

The amount of sodium you lose in sweat depends upon how acclimated you are to exercising in the heat. At the beginning of the summer, your sweat is far saltier than at the end of the season. As you adjust to exercising in the heat, you sweat less salt. Training itself also produces changes in sweat gland function, resulting in the production of more dilute sweat. Nature protects you from the potential dangers of becoming salt depleted!

Athletes who eat a low-salt diet tend to have low-salt sweat. The less salt that you eat, the less you'll lose. The kidneys and sweat glands tend to conserve sodium when it's in short supply.

Sports Drinks

Many athletes are confused by the vast array of sports drinks— Gatorade, Exceed, Max, and other fluid replacers with electrolytes, glucose, or glucose polymers. They want to know if these products are helpful, or if water is best. Water will always be an excellent fluid replacer. It's what your body needs. It's inexpensive, readily available, and popular. It's absorbed quickly and does a fine job. Water works well for most recreational athletes, especially in combination with an appropriate sports diet.

If you're running a marathon, competing in a triathlon, or participating in some high-intensity endurance event that lasts longer than 90 minutes, you might want a beverage that contains a small amount of sugar to improve your stamina. Unlike sugar taken before exercise, which might result in subsequent low blood sugar, sugar taken during exercise can enhance performance because the body does not secrete insulin during exercise (see chapter 4).

During a moderate-to-hard endurance workout, carbohydrates supply about 50 percent of the energy. As you deplete carbohydrates from muscle glycogen stores, you increasingly rely on blood sugar for energy. By consuming carbohydrates that help maintain a normal blood sugar level, you can exercise for a longer time. Also, much of your endurance capacity depends upon your mental stamina. Maintaining a normal blood sugar level will help you to concentrate.

The muscles in a 150-pound cyclist can use blood glucose at the rate of about 1 gram (4 calories) of carbohydrates for every minute of hard exercise. Theoretically, a similar-size athlete should try to consume 60 grams (240 calories) per hour of endurance exercise; this is the equivalent of about 5 cups of Gatorade, 3 cups of Exceed, 2-1/4 cups of sugar-sweetened soft drinks, or 2-1/4 cups of slightly diluted juices that offer about 100 calories per 8 ounces. That breaks down into 60 calories every 15 minutes. This is more than most athletes are likely to consume, but it emphasizes the importance of experimenting with ''carbo-hydration'' during your endurance training to determine how much you can tolerate and which fluids work best for you.

Thanks to the power of the media, commercial sports drinks are being perceived as the athlete's "edge" when it comes to fluid replacements. Although the advertisements may lead you to believe that these special formulations are the ultimate in carbohydration, keep in mind that successful athletes have been drinking home-made sports drinks for years:

- Cyclists religiously fill water bottles with tea with honey.
- Marathoners plant friends along the race-route to hand them defizzed cola.
- Cross-country skiers welcome warm blueberry soup or other sugar solutions at feed stations.

Commercial fluid replacers are nutritionally similar to diluted soft drinks but more expensive. They offer carbohydrates (about 50 to 70 calories per cup), insignificant amounts of sodium and potassium, and generally little or no other nutritional value. During a 2-hour workout burning 1,000 calories, it is possible to lose 180 milligrams of potassium and 1,000 milligrams of sodium. These minerals are not replaced by fluid replacers.

Most fluid replacers are purposely designed to be very weak solutions that can be quickly assimilated by your body during exercise. The caloric content of a beverage exerts control over how fast a liquid empties from the stomach into the intestine, where it enters into the blood stream and becomes available to replace sweat losses. If a drink is highly concentrated, it's likely to take longer to empty from the stomach than a fluid replacer.

I often talk to cyclists who not only drink a fluid replacer but simultaneously snack on granola bars and bananas. These foods negate the purpose of the fluid replacer because the high caloric density of the snack delays gastric emptying. Solid foods take longer to empty from the stomach than fluids; high-calorie foods and fluids take longer to empty than lower calorie choices. Fluid replacers are dilute beverages designed for highly competitive athletes who prefer to only drink during the event.

The best time to drink fluid replacers is during exercise:

- *Not* 20 to 45 minutes beforehand, when they might trigger a hypoglycemic reaction.
- *Not* afterwards, when your muscles want full-strength, carbohydrate-rich beverages to replace the glycogen burned during the event and the minerals lost in sweat (see Table 10.3).

Glucose polymers are short chains of glucose molecules. They have become popular with endurance athletes who want carbohydrates that

Table 10.3 Fluid Replacers

Drink	Calories per 8 oz	Potassium (mg) per 8 oz	Sodium (mg) per 8 oz
Gatorade	50	25	110
Recharge	50	25	15
Vitalade	85	90	—
Exceed	70	45	50
Coke	95	—	8
Pepsi	100	8	6
Orange juice	110	475	2
Apple juice	115	300	5
Cranberry juice	150	60	10
Grape juice	155	335	5
Cranapple	175	70	5
Orange, lg	120	440	0
Fruit yogurt	225	400	120
Possible losses in a 2-hour workout:	1,000 calories	180 mg potassium	1,000 mg sodium

Note. Nutrient data from *Bowes and Church's Food Values of Portions Commonly Used* (14th ed.) by J. Pennington and H. Church, 1985, Philadelphia: Lippincott. Adapted by permission.

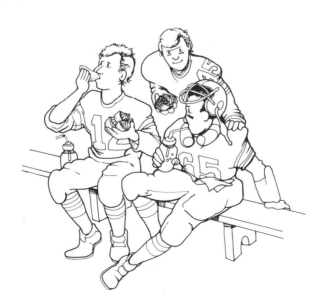

settle comfortably and leave the stomach quickly, but who don't want to drink very sweet liquids or eat solid foods.

The verdict is still unclear as to whether a marathoner, triathlete, or other endurance athlete will perform better with a traditional sugared drink (defizzed coke, tea with honey), a polymer drink, or plain water with snacks. The bottom line depends on the intensity of the sport and what works best for that individual's body. Some endurance athletes still feel safest with plain water; it's tried and true. Others prefer a particular brand of sports drink. Some prefer diluted apple juice or orange sections plus water. You have to experiment to determine what works best for you.

CHAPTER 11

Protein and Performance

Traditionally, athletes have devoured platefuls of beef, eggs, tuna, chicken, and other proteins—the theory being that if you eat a lot of protein, you'll build a lot of muscle.

But extra protein does not build muscle bulk; exercise does. To build and strengthen muscles, you have to include resistance exercise, such as weight lifting, in your workout program.

For you to have enough energy for muscle-building exercise, your diet should be about 60 percent carbohydrate and 15 percent protein. Strange as it may sound, body builders and marathon runners can eat the same foods. Body builders tend to have comparatively more muscle mass than runners, and they generally eat more calories:

- A 150-pound runner might eat 2,600 calories:

    15% x 2,600 = 390 protein calories,

- whereas a 200-pound body builder might eat 3,600 calories:

    15% x 3,600 = 540 protein calories.

Mike, a national-class power lifter, was very confused by conflicting stories about the best foods for building muscles. His buddies at the gym would tell him to bulk-up on steak, tuna, turkey, and egg whites—and to guzzle protein drinks. But his neighbor, a marathon runner, encouraged him to carbo-load with lots of spaghetti. Mike's mother, an Italian, fed him what she thought was best—pasta. I reassured Mike that pasta was indeed the better choice to combine with his training program. He exclaimed, "I knew that pasta helped me to become a winner!"

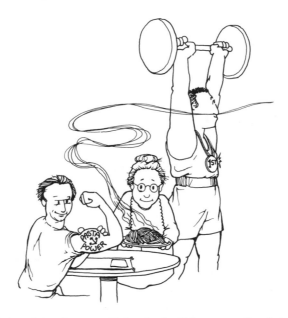

As I explained in chapter 7, body builders need a lot of carbohydrates because these nutrients are stored in the muscles for energy. You can't lift weights and demand a lot from your workout sessions if your muscles are carbohydrate-depleted. Protein-based diets don't provide muscle fuel and won't let you exercise hard enough to build to your potential.

The best sports diet contains adequate, but not excess, protein—to build and repair muscle tissue, to grow hair and fingernails, to produce hormones, and to replace red blood cells. Most athletes who eat small to moderate portions of protein-rich foods daily get at least twice the protein they need; any excess protein is simply stored as fat.

How Much Protein Do You Need?

When it comes to protein intake, athletes seem to fall into two categories:

1. *Protein pushers*—the body builders, weight lifters, football players who think they can't get enough of the stuff.
2. *Protein avoiders*—the runners, triathletes, dancers who never touch meat, and who trade most protein calories for more carbohydrates.

Both groups may perform poorly due to dietary inbalances. Doug, for example, was a protein pusher. A high school football player, he routinely snacked after practice on a few large burgers and a quart of milk. That one snack satisfied his protein needs for the whole day! As an athlete, he had a slightly higher protein need than a sedentary person, but he overcompensated for that need with the big portions he devoured at meals alone, never mind his high-protein snack.

John, a proud triathlete who boasted about his high-carbohydrate, low-fat, low-protein diet, was a protein avoider. He was humbled upon learning that his food intake was deficient not only in protein, but also in iron, zinc, calcium, and several other nutrients. No wonder he became anemic, suffered a lingering cold and flu, and performed poorly despite consistent training (see Table 11.1 for a sample of a protein-deficient sports diet).

Research has yet to define the exact protein needs of sports-active people because their needs vary. People who probably need more

Table 11.1 Protein Deficiency in a High-Carbohydrate Sports Diet

Many athletes eat too many carbohydrates and neglect their protein needs—0.6 to 0.9 grams of protein per pound of body weight, or roughly the equivalent of 15 percent of total daily calories. The following is a typical example of a protein-deficient diet of 3,000 calories per day. Only 6.5 percent of the calories are from protein, which translates to 0.3 grams of protein per pound, or no more than half the recommended intake.

Meal	Protein (g)	Approximate calories
Breakfast		
2 bagels	4	400
2 c orange juice	2	220
Lunch		
2 lg bananas	3	300
2 c apple juice	—	240
1 lg muffin	4	300
Dinner		
3 c cooked pasta	20	660
1 c tomato sauce	2	100
2 c cranberry juice	—	300
Snack		
1 c dried fruit	5	480
Total	42	3,000
Recommended intake	90-135	

protein per pound of body weight than the current RDA of 0.4 grams include these:

- Endurance athletes and others doing intense exercise
- Dieters consuming too few calories
- Untrained people beginning an exercise program

Here are some safe recommendations for protein intake:

	Grams of protein/pound body weight
Sedentary adult	0.4
Active adult	0.4-0.6
Growing athlete	0.6-0.9
Adult building muscle mass	0.6-0.9

Calculating Your Needs

It's easy to figure out your protein needs and if you're meeting them in your current diet. Here's how:

First, identify yourself in the categories listed in the preceding protein-intake chart, which includes a margin of safety for growing individuals and those building muscle mass. Then multiply your weight (in pounds) by the number for your category to yield the number of grams of protein you need each day.

A 120-pound, athletic women, for example, categorized as an "active adult," would need about 72 grams of protein per day:

$$120 \text{ lb} \times 0.6 \text{ g/lb} = 72 \text{ g protein}$$

A 150-pound teenage swimmer in the category of "growing athlete," would need about 135 grams of protein per day:

$$150 \text{ lb} \times 0.9 \text{ g/lb} = 135 \text{ g protein}$$

Keeping track of your protein intake is easy; all it takes is a little time. List everything you eat and drink for one 24-hour period (you can do this over a period of days if you want to get a more accurate picture of your overall diet). Then use the nutrition information on food labels to start a tally of the protein you consumed. For example, a 6.5-ounce can of tuna might tell you it contains 25 grams of protein per serving and 2 servings per can. So, if you ate the whole can of tuna, you got 50 grams of protein.

Here's a list of the protein amounts in some foods that are often unlabeled or lack labels with nutrient information:

Item*	Serving size	Protein (g)
Meat, poultry, fish	3 oz cooked**	21
Beans, dried peas, lentils	1/2 c cooked	7
Egg	1 large	7
Peas, carrots, beets	1/2 c cooked	2
Potato	1 small	2

The rule of thumb for getting adequate, but not excess, protein in your diet is to include 2 cups of low-fat milk or yogurt plus 4 to 6 ounces of protein-rich foods per day. Combined with the small amounts of protein in other foods that round out the meals, this should suit the needs of a healthy adult. Growing teens should drink an additional 2 cups of milk. Here's a sample of one day's worth of protein foods for a healthy, active adult:

Breakfast: 1 c milk on cereal

Lunch: 2 oz protein sandwich filling (tuna, roast beef, turkey); 1 c yogurt

Dinner: 4 oz meat, fish, poultry, or the equivalent in lentils or other beans and legumes (1/2 c beans is equivalent to approximately 1 oz of animal protein).

Of course, you need to eat other foods to round out your nutritional requirements!

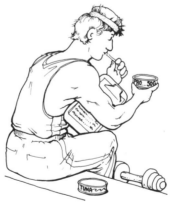

*Most fruits, vegetables, and juices provide well under 1 gram of protein per serving, which, depending on how much you eat, might contribute a total of 5 to 10 grams per day. Butter, margarine, oil, sugar, candy, soda, alcohol, coffee, and tea contain no protein, and desserts contain very little.

**3 oz cooked meat is about 4 oz raw (about the size of a woman's palm).

Problems With Too Much Protein

Luke, an aspiring basketball champ, called himself a meat-and-potatoes man. He'd chow down on burgers and thick steaks and barely nibble on the spuds, much to the detriment of his athletic aspirations. He tired easily and asked me if this high-protein diet might be hurting his performance. Here's what I told him:

• If you fill your stomach with protein, you won't be fueling your muscles with carbohydrates.

• Anyone who eats excess protein may need to urinate more frequently, because protein breaks down into urea, a waste product eliminated in the urine. Frequent toilet trips may be an inconvenience during training and competition, to say nothing of increasing the risk of becoming dehydrated and burdening the kidneys.

• You can save money by reducing larger-than-necessary portions of animal proteins (beef, lamb, pork, fish) and use it to purchase more carbohydrates, such as potatoes, grains, fruits, and vegetables.

• A diet high in protein is often also high in fat (greasy burgers, bacon, fat-marbled meats, fried chicken, and so on). For both your heart's sake and for improved athletic performance, you should reduce your intake of the saturated fats often found in animal proteins.

I encouraged Luke to reduce his meat portions at dinner to one third of his plate and to fill two thirds of it with potatoes, vegetables, and bread. Within 2 days he noticed an improvement in his energy level. He then changed his breakfast from steak and eggs to cereal and bananas, and lunch became chili or pasta or casseroles rather than

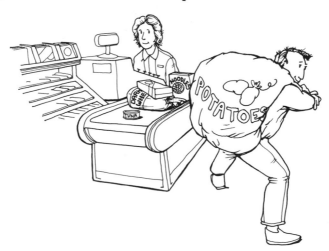

burgers. His diet gradually became a winner. "You know," he now says, "food works. The right foods definitely enhance my sports performance!"

Protein and the Vegetarian

Most people who call themselves vegetarians make the effort to include in their daily diets plant proteins, such as peanut butter, sunflower seeds, tofu, and beans. Some non–meat eaters, however, fuel up on carbohydrates and neglect their protein needs. A typical protein-deficient intake would look like this:

Breakfast: bran muffins and juice

Lunch: dried fruit and a bagel

Snack: rice cakes and juice

Dinner: pasta with tomato sauce and a salad

Whatever their reasons for abstaining from meat, some vegetarians overlook the fact that they still need to eat enough protein to maintain good health.

Female athletes often fit into this non–meat-eater category. Sue, now a healthy dancer, used to live on fruit for breakfast, a salad for lunch, and stir-fried vegetables with brown rice for dinner. She thought her diet was great when in fact it was deficient in several nutrients. At one point she suffered a stress fracture that healed very slowly. She had spindly arms and legs—the "anorexic look"—and her menstrual period was absent, another sign of an unhealthy body related to her protein- and nutrient-deficient diet. Current research suggests that amenorrhea puts a woman at a risk 4.5 times higher than normal for suffering a stress fracture (Nelson, 1986; Clark, 1988).

The Right Combinations

If you want to omit animal protein from your diet, or you already do, then you need to know how to combine vegetable and other proteins in the right amounts to be sure that you are getting enough high-quality protein each day.

All proteins are made up of *amino acids*, which your body uses to build tissue; hence their nickname, "building blocks." There are 22 of these amino acids, and every protein in your body is made up of some combination of them. Your body can synthesize some amino acids itself; 9 of them, however, called the *essential* amino acids, must come from the foods you eat.

Animal protein contains all of the essential amino acids and is often referred to as "complete" protein. The protein in vegetables and other sources is "incomplete" because it does not contain all of the essential amino acids. Thus, vegetarians must understand how to combine incomplete proteins to make them complete. The following combinations do the job:

Grains + milk products (for less-strict vegetarians)
    cereal + milk
    pasta + cheese
    bread + cheese

Grains + beans and legumes (such as peanuts and kidney, pinto, lima, and navy beans)
    rice + beans
    croutons + split-pea soup
    tortillas + beans
    corn bread + chili beans
    brown bread + baked beans

Legumes + seeds
    chick-peas + tahini (as in hummus)
    tofu + sesame seeds

Following these guidelines, vegetarian athletes can plan their diets to be sure they consume an adequate amount of complete protein every day. Table 11.2 gives a sample meal plan for a vegetarian who requires approximately 2,800 calories per day.

The same folks who avoid red meat for health reasons often turn to eggs and cheese for protein. They thrive on buttery omelets, rice casseroles smothered with cream sauces, or salads and whole grain breads piled high with cheese. They're unaware, though, that cheese and eggs have far more fat and/or cholesterol than lean meats, and that a grilled cheese or egg salad sandwich is, in that respect, worse than a lean roast beef sandwich without mayonnaise. Refer to Table 2.4, page 34, for amount of fat and cholesterol in some foods.

Even though vegetarians can get the right protein in adequate amounts, many lack iron and zinc, minerals found primarily in meats and other animal products. Iron is a vital component in red blood cells, and zinc plays an important role in tissue growth and maintenance. Chapter 12 explains how vegetarians and meat eaters alike can ensure a proper intake of these two nutrients.

Table 11.2   Sample Menu for a Sports-Active Vegetarian

Meal	Protein (g)	Calories
Breakfast		
1 c orange juice	2	110
2 c bran flakes	8	240
1 med banana	1	100
1-1/2 c milk	12	150
Lunch		
2 peanut butter sandwiches*	30	700
1 apple	1	100
2 c milk	16	200
Snack		
1 c fruit yogurt	10	250
Dinner		
1 med pizza	70	1,000
Total	150	2,850

*(2 T peanut butter on each).

Protein Supplements and Amino Acids

According to the advertisements in body-building magazines, protein powders and amino acid pills are essential for optimal muscle development. If you've been hanging around the power gyms, you've undoubtedly heard intense conversations about some of these products, such as arginine, ornithine, and free-form amino acids. The protein-praising body builders who come to me for advice often lug gym bags bulging with assorted pills, powders, and potions. They wonder if these supplements are worth the price and if they work. Some are avid believers in the stuff, and others are skeptical.

If you're struggling to develop bigger muscles and improve your strength, you'll get more value from the following tips than from a canister of special supplements:

- Exercise, not extra protein, is the key to developing bigger muscles.
- You may be consuming excessive calories in your effort to eat excessive protein. Your body will burn very small amounts, but most of it will be converted to fat and stored in adipose tissue.

- The amount of protein or amino acids in expensive powders and pills is less than that which you might easily get from foods. For example, you have to eat 5 tablespoons of one popular protein powder at a cost of $1.10 to get the same amount of protein as that in a 3-1/2-ounce can of tuna at about half the price. See Table 11.3 for more comparisons.

The next chapter provides more detail on different types of nutrition supplements.

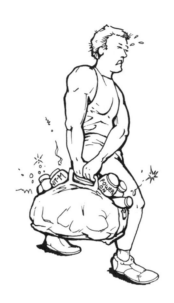

Table 11.3 Amino Acids: Food Versus Pills

This table compares the milligrams of two amino acids as available in food and in several popular protein supplements. The second part lists the approximate cost for 25 grams of protein.

Food or protein Supplement	Amount	Arginine (mg)	Tryptophan (mg)	Amount needed for 25 g protein	Approximate cost ($)
Chicken breast	4 oz (raw)	2,100	400	3 oz (cooked)	.30
Eggs	2	780	200	4	.35
Skim milk	1 c	300	120	3 c	.55
Amino Fuel	1 svg	120	75	7 wafers	1.45
Coach's Formula	1 svg	410	170	5 T	1.10
Dynamic Muscle	1 svg	680	240	4 T	.70

Note. Nutrient data from *Bowes and Church's Food Values of Portions Commonly Used* (14th ed.) by J. Pennington and H. Church, 1985, Philadelphia: Lippincott. Adapted by permission. Protein supplement data from labels.

CHAPTER 12

Supplements: What They Are, What They Aren't

The supplement business is big business! Approximately 40 percent of Americans take supplements. A higher percentage of athletes take them. Among the nation's top female runners, 91 percent reported taking supplements on a regular basis (Stewart, 1985; Clark, 1988).

Advertisements have convinced many people that they need to supplement their diets. As one working mother claims, "I don't have time to eat right, so I take supplements to compensate for my poor eating habits." A squash player and banker reports, "I think of vitamins as health insurance that helps protect me from stress." A triathlete and construction worker expresses concern about the nutritional quality of his food choices: "I'm so active, I must need more vitamins than my fast-food diet can provide."

Being constantly under stress, grabbing hit-or-miss meals, juggling work with workouts, and demanding intense physical efforts from their muscles, these active folks have turned to a potential panacea—vitamin supplements: a super-sports pack with each meal, jumbo pills after every weight workout, vitamin C after every cough.

Pill pushers insistently claim that supplements are necessary to guard your health, compensate for processed foods, enhance your athletic abilities, and promote future "super health." However, the same ads and salespeople that entice you to take supplements neglect to mention that you still need to eat well, regardless of the number of pills you pop.

Vitamin Supplements

Too many people appeal to their vitamin-pill breakfasts to rationalize their chocolate chip cookie lunches. They naively believe that a vitamin supplement satisfies 100 percent of their nutritional needs. They're wrong. They may get 100 percent of their *vitamin* needs at breakfast, but we need not only vitamins, but also protein, minerals, energy, and fiber (see the following chart). No vitamin provides energy (calories) or compensates for a lunch of sugars and fats.

The Fundamental 40 Nutrients

1 *Carbohydrates*

9 *Protein* (9 essential amino acids):
histidine	phenylalanine
isoleucine	threonine
leucine	tryptophan
lysine	valine
methionine	

1 *Fat* (1 essential fatty acid):
linoleic acid

13 *Vitamins* (4 fat-soluble):
A, D, E, K

Vitamins (9 water-soluble):
B_1 (thiamin)	folacin
B_2 (riboflavin)	biotin
B_6 (pyridoxine)	pantothenic acid
niacin	C (ascorbic acid)
B_{12}	

12 *Minerals* (3 major):
calcium
phosphorous
magnesium

Minerals (9 trace):
iron	fluoride
zinc	chromium
iodine	selenium
copper	molybdenum
manganese	

(Cont.)

3   *Electrolytes*
   sodium
   potassium
   chloride

1   *Water*
_____

40   Total

Other substances that are presently being studied to determine possible human requirements:

aluminum	nickel
arsenic	silicon
boron	strontium
cadmium	titanium
choline	tin
cobalt	vanadium

By eating a variety of foods from the four food groups, you will get the fundamental 40 nutrients required by the body to maintain good health.

_____

Note. Reprinted from "Recommended Dietary Allowances," 9th revised edition, 1980, with permission of the National Academy Press, Washington, DC.

_____

Q. *What are vitamins?*

A. Vitamins are metabolic catalysts that regulate biochemical reactions within your body. Your body cannot manufacture them, which is why you must obtain them through your diet. To date, 13 vitamins have been discovered, each with a specific function. For example, thiamin helps convert glucose into energy, vitamin D controls the way your body uses calcium, and vitamin A is part of an eye pigment that helps you see in the dim light. Refer to Table 12.1 for more detailed information on vitamins.

You need adequate vitamins to function optimally, but an excess offers no competitive edge. No scientific evidence to date proves that extra vitamins enhance performance. Despite claims to the contrary, supplements will not

- enhance performance,
- increase strength or endurance,
- prevent injuries or illness,
- provide energy, or
- build muscles.

Table 12.1 Vitamin Breakdown

Vitamin	US RDA	Functions	Sources
A (retinol)	5,000 IU	Helps maintain eyes, skin, linings of the nose, mouth, digestive, and urinary tracts.	Liver, whole milk, butter, cheese, fortified margarine, carrots, spinach
Thiamin (B₁)	1.5 mg	Helps convert carbohydrates into energy.	Yeast, rice, whole grain breads and cereals, liver, pork, poultry, eggs, fish, fruits, and vegetables
Riboflavin (B₂)	1.7 mg	Helps energy release; helps maintain skin, mucous membranes, and nervous structures.	Dairy products, liver, yeast, fruits, whole grain breads and cereals, vegetables, lean meats, poultry
Niacin (B₃)	20 mg	Helps convert carbohydrates, fats, and protein into energy; essential for growth; aids synthesis of hormones.	Liver, chicken, turkey, halibut, tuna, milk, eggs, grains, fruits and vegetables, enriched breads and cereals
B₆ (pyridoxine, pyridoxamine)	2.0 mg	Aids in more than 60 enzyme reactions.	Milk, liver, lean meats, whole grain breads and cereals, vegetables
Folic acid	0.4 mg	Aids blood-cell production; helps maintain nervous system.	Liver, many vegetables

(Cont.)

Table 12.1 (Continued)

Vitamin	US RDA	Functions	Sources
Biotin	0.3 mg	Aids in intermediary metabolism of carbohydrates, fats, and protein.	Widely distributed in foods.
Pantothenic acid	10 mg	Aids in metabolism of carbohydrates, fats, and protein.	Eggs, liver, kidneys, peanuts, whole grains, most vegetables, fish
B$_{12}$	6.0 mcg	Helps synthesize red and white blood cells; aids many metabolic reactions.	Liver, meat, eggs, milk
C (ascorbic acid)	60 mg	Helps maintain and repair connective tissue, bones, teeth, cartilage; promotes healing.	Broccoli, brussels sprouts, citrus fruits, and vegetables
D (cholecalciferol)	400 IU	Helps regulate calcium and phosphorus metabolism; essential for bones and teeth.	Fortified milk, fish-liver oils; sunlight on skin produces vitamin D
E (tocopherol)	30 IU	Protects and maintains cellular membranes.	Vegetable oils, whole grains, leafy vegetables
K	70 to 140 mcg	Used in synthesis of prothrombin (essential for blood clotting).	Green leafy vegetables, soybeans, beef liver, widespread in foods

Copyright 1986 by Consumers Union of United State, Inc., Mount Vernon, NY 10553. Reprinted by permission from *Consumer Reports*, March 1986.

Granted, if you have a vitamin deficiency that is impairing your performance, a supplement can correct that problem. However, vitamin deficiencies are generally related to a larger medical problem that needs attention, such as anorexia, unhealthful weight reduction, poor eating habits, or malabsorption problems.

Q. *Does exercise increase vitamin needs?*

A. No. Exercising doesn't burn vitamins, just as cars don't burn spark plugs. Vitamins are catalysts that are needed for metabolic processes to occur. There is no evidence to date that vitamin supplementation improves performance in nutritionally adequate people.

Recent studies suggest that the established RDAs for some vitamins may be too low for active people. For instance, for riboflavin (vitamin B_2, important for converting food into energy), the current RDA of 0.6 milligrams per 1,000 calories may be inadequate for active people; 1.1 milligrams might be a better dose. In these studies, supplements did not enhance exercise performance (Belko, 1987). However, you don't need to rush out and buy riboflavin. You can easily meet your need for riboflavin at breakfast with cereal with milk! The increased requirement is far less than you might think and athletes who eat decently are unlikely to suffer deficiencies of riboflavin or other vitamins.

The RDAs are not a minimal requirement. They include about a 30-percent margin of safety to cover the nutritional needs of 97 percent of healthy Americans, including those with higher than average needs. You can meet these needs, even if you're eating on the run, by choosing a variety of wholesome foods from the four food groups.

Athletes generally consume more food, and therein more vitamins, than inactive folks with smaller appetites. Deficiencies are less likely to occur in a sports-active person with a ravenous appetite than in a sedentary person who nibbles at morsels.

Q. *Is a daily supplement good health insurance for the days I eat poorly?*

A. If you usually eat a well-balanced diet, a supplement is unnecessary for that occasional day when all good intentions get waylaid. Pat, a 46-year-old golfer and office manager, ate a well-balanced diet 6 out of 7 days a week. Fridays were her downfall because of fatigue and work stress. She'd inevitably ''go off the deep end'' and comfort herself with donuts, french fries, and ice cream, and take megadoses of vitamin supplements to protect against nutritional deficiencies.

I assured Pat that a nutritional deficiency would not develop overnight. She could survive on less than a daily 100 percent of every vitamin because she stored vitamins in her body, some in stockpiles (A, D, E, K—the fat-soluble vitamins) and others in smaller amounts (B, C—the water-soluble vitamins). Like most healthy people, she probably

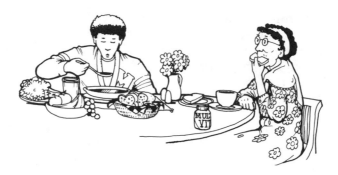

had enough vitamin C stored in her liver to last 6 weeks. One day of decadent eating would not have resulted in a nutritionally unsound body. Nutritional deficiencies generally develop over the course of months or years.

Supplements for Special Situations?

Q. *Should anyone take vitamin supplements?*

A. Although I always advise athletes to get their vitamins from wholesome foods, I do recommend a simple multivitamin supplement for some individuals at risk of nutritional deficiencies. Supplements can be appropriate for people who have the following characteristics:

Restricting Calories.   Dieters who eat less than 1,200 to 1,500 calories daily may miss out on some important nutrients.

Energy Efficient.   Some individuals consume far fewer calories than they deserve—hence far fewer vitamins. This commonly happens with chronic dieters, formerly obese people who are currently abnormally thin, and those who exercise excessively.

Allergic to Certain Foods.   People who can't eat certain types of foods, such as fruits or wheat, need to compensate with alternative sources to avoid deficiencies in some nutrients.

Lactose Intolerant.   This is an inability to digest milk sugar, common among blacks and Hispanics. Dairy foods are the best source riboflavin and calcium.

Pregnant.   Expectant mothers require additional vitamins, but they should consult their physicians before taking a supplement.

Total Vegetarians.   People who completely abstain from eating animal foods may become deficient in vitamins B$_{12}$, D, and riboflavin.

Vitamins as Health Insurance

Q. *Are supplements good health insurance?*

A. When it comes to nourishing your body, I always recommend that you get the vitamins you need from the food you eat; food first. If for psychological "health insurance" you wish to supplement your diet, you can take a single one-a-day-type multivitamin if you like.

Usually, people who care enough to take supplements are the ones least likely to need them! However, some folks take supplements as an alternative to making responsible food choices. In one of my workshops for aerobic dancers, almost half of the dancers reported taking supplements to compensate for poor dietary habits. Other reasons for taking supplements include hit-or-miss eating, chronic stress, fast foods, crash diets, and inadequate sleep. In my opinion, it is naive to think that a pill of any type can magically compensate for an erosive lifestyle.

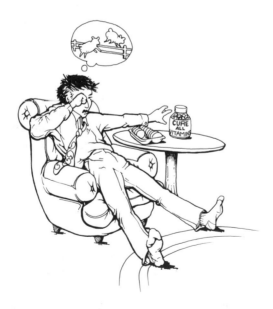

Many athletes who prescribe supplements for themselves have little knowledge of how vitamins work or what doses are appropriate. They figure that if a little bit is good, then a lot must be better. These athletes do an excellent job of supporting the vitamin industry and may also be setting themselves up for toxic reactions. For example, high doses of vitamin B_6 (greater than 1.0 gram per day over a period of months) may cause numbness, loss of muscle coordination, and paralysis; too much vitamin C (more than 1 gram per day) may lead to intestinal problems, kidney stones, and diarrhea. In general, any dose greater than 10 times the RDA is considered a "megadose" and should be taken only under a physician's guidance.

If you are currently taking supplements and are not knowledgeable about vitamins, I recommend that you get a nutrition checkup with a registered dietitian (RD). You will be able to evaluate your diet and learn not only what nutrients you are getting, but also the best food sources for those that you're missing. To find an RD, ask your doctor for a referral, call the nutrition department at your local hospital or sports medicine clinic, or look in the yellow pages under "Dietitian" and select a name followed by "RD."

Some sophisticated supplement users do not think of vitamins as compensating for dietary inadequacies, but rather view them as therapeutic agents that might enhance future longevity. Because many diseases of aging are affected by diet, these health-conscious folks not only eat wisely but also take supplements to complement their total health program. See chapter 2 for a discussion of this issue in relation to cancer, or read some of the books listed in Appendix B.

Minerals

Minerals are present in all living cells. They occur freely in nature in the soil and water and travel through the food chain by being absorbed into the plants that grow in the soil and then into the animals that consume the plants and water. Vegetables of the same species can differ in mineral content, depending on the soil in which they were grown.

Each mineral has a unique role in the body. For instance, calcium maintains the rigid structure of the bones, potassium and sodium control water balance in the body, iron assists with oxygen transport, and magnesium activates enzymes and is required for muscular contraction.

You need some minerals in large amounts: sodium, potassium, chloride, calcium, phosphorus,and magnesium. Others, such as iron, zinc, selenium, and iodine, are needed in smaller amounts. As with vitamins, you can get the minerals you need if you eat a variety of wholesome foods. Iron and zinc can be exceptions to that general rule, particularly for those who abstain from red meat; the same is true of calcium for those who abstain from dairy products.

Iron

Iron is a necessary component of hemoglobin, the protein that transports oxygen from the lungs to the working muscles. If you are iron deficient, you're likely to fatigue easily upon exertion. Athletes at highest risk of suffering from iron deficiency anemia include

- female athletes who lose iron through menstrual bleeding;
- athletes who eat no red meat (the best dietary sources of iron);
- marathon runners, who may damage red blood cells by pounding their feet on the ground during training;
- endurance athletes, who may lose significant amounts of iron through heavy sweat losses; and
- teenage athletes who are growing quickly and may consume inadequate iron to meet their expanded requirements.

Follow these tips to help you boost your iron intake.

1.   Eat *lean* cuts of beef, lamb, and pork, and the dark meat of chicken or turkey, 3 to 4 times per week.

2.   Select breads and cereals with the words "iron-enriched" or "fortified" on the label. This added iron supplements the small amount that naturally occurs in grains. Eat these foods with a source of vitamin C (for example, orange juice with cereal, tomato on a sandwich) to enhance iron absorption.

3.   Use cast-iron skillets for cooking. They offer more nutritional value than stainless steel cookware! The iron content of spaghetti sauce simmered in a cast-iron skillet for 3 hours may increase from 3 to 88 milligrams for each half-cup of sauce.

4.   Abstain from consistently drinking coffee or tea with all meals, particularly if you're prone to being anemic. Substances in these beverages can interfere with iron absorption.

5.   Combine poorly absorbed vegetarian sources of iron (10-percent absorption rate) with animal sources (40-percent absorption rate). For example, eat broccoli with beef, spinach with chicken, chili with lean hamburger, and lentil soup with turkey.

For a list of foods highest in iron, refer to Table 12.2.

Zinc

The mineral zinc is a part of more than 100 enzymes that make your body function properly. For example, it helps remove carbon dioxide from your muscles when you exercise. Zinc also enhances the healing process.

Table 12.2   Iron in Foods

The RDA for iron is 10 milligrams for men and 18 milligrams for women. This target intake is set high because iron is poorly absorbed. The best iron sources are from animal products.

Food sources	Iron (mg)	Food sources	Iron (mg)
Animal			
Liver, 4 oz cooked	10*	Baked beans, 1/2 c	2
Beef, 4 oz roasted	6*	Kidney beans, 1/2 c	2
Pork, 4 oz roasted	5*	Bean curd, 1/4 cake	2
Turkey, 4 oz roasted dark			
meat	3*	**Grains**	
Tuna, 6.5 oz light	2*	Cereal, 100% fortified, 3/4 c	18
Chicken breast, 4 oz	1*	Kellogg's Raisin Bran, 1/2 c	18
Fish, 4 oz broiled			
haddock	1*	Cream of Wheat	9
Egg, 1 lg	1	Wheat Chex, 2/3 c	4.5
Fruits		Spaghetti, 1/2 c cooked,	
Prune juice, 8 oz	3	enriched	1
Apricots, 12 halves dried	2	Bread, 1 sl enriched	1
Dates, 10 dried	1	**Other**	
Raisins, 1/3 c	1	Molasses, 1 T blackstrap	2
Vegetables/legumes		Brewer's yeast, 1 T	2
Spinach, 1/2 c cooked	2	Wheat germ, 1/4 cup	2
Green peas, 1/2 c cooked	1		
Broccoli, 1/2 c cooked	1		

* This iron is best absorbed.

Because the zinc in animal protein is absorbed better than that from plants, vegetarian athletes are at risk of having a zinc deficiency. For a list of foods rich in zinc, refer to Table 12.3.

Other Pills and Potions

Sports enthusiasts typically yearn to improve athletic performance effortlessly, without sweat! Many hopeful folks look for magic pills and potions that just may offer that winner's edge.

They swallow the advertising claims that promise bulging biceps, endless energy, and faster feet. Unfortunately, they don't realize that if a claim sounds too good to be true, it probably is.

Table 12.3 Zinc in Foods

The RDA for zinc is 15 milligrams. This recommended intake is set high and may be hard to consume, but it should be a target intake, particularly for athletes who sweat heavily and may incur subsequent zinc losses.

Animal sources	Zinc (mg)	Vegetarian sources	Zinc (mg)
Beef, steak, 4 oz	7	Almonds, 1 oz	0.7
Beef, liver, 4 oz	6	Cashews, 6–8	0.6
Chicken leg, 4 oz	3.5	Peanut butter, 1 T	0.5
Chicken breast, 4 oz	1		
Chicken liver, 4 oz	4	Garbanzo beans, 1 c	2
Pork, 4 oz	4.5	Lentils, 1 c	2
Turkey leg, 4 oz	5	Bread, white, 1 sl	0.2
Turkey breast, 4 oz	2	Bread, whole wheat, 1 sl	0.5
Cheese, cheddar, 1 oz	1	Rice, white, 1 c	0.6
Cheese, cottage, 1 c	1	Rice, brown, 1 c	1.2
Milk, 1 c	1	Oatmeal, 1 c	1.2
Yogurt, 1 c	1	40% Bran flakes, 1 oz	1
		Wheat germ, 1/4 c	3.2
Egg, 1 lg	0.5	Shredded wheat, 1 oz	0.8
Clams, 4–5	1	Apple, med	0.1
Crab, 1 c	6.5	Banana, 1 med	0.3
Fish, white, 4 oz	1	Raisins, 1/4 c	0.1
Oysters, 2–4	75		
Tuna, 1 can (6.5 oz)	2	Potato, med boiled	0.3
		Spinach, 1 c raw	0.5

Note. Nutrient data from *Bowes and Church's Food Values of Portions Commonly Used* (14th ed.) by J. Pennington and H. Church, 1985, Philadelphia: Lippincott. Adapted by permission.

There's only one way to improve performance: You have to train hard and eat properly. However, hocus pocus thrives among ever-hopeful sports-active people of all ages and abilities.

- Beginners want a pill that will help them be stronger in 1 day.
- Experienced competitors want a potion that will shave seconds off their performance times.

For a price, you can buy any variety of assorted athletes' formulas that supposedly will make you a winner.

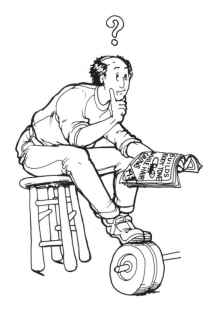

No scientific data, to date, supports any of the intriguing claims.

- Protein supplements don't build muscles.
- Bee pollen has no energy-enhancing effect.
- Ginseng won't make you faster.
- Spirulina isn't the final cure for aches and injuries.

Peter, a body builder, swore by the eight dessicated liver pills he managed to choke down each day after his workout. He felt certain they helped his lifting. I doubt it. The amount of liver he actually consumed was less than an ounce, an amount that would barely nourish an infant, to say nothing of a hulk! But Peter believed those pills were energizers, so they probably were for him. See chapter 11 for more information about protein supplements.

If special pills and potions improve performance, it's undoubtedly because the athlete believes they will help. Your mind is very powerful and can elicit from you performances that may be far beyond your expectations. This is called the *placebo effect*. Yet, if you happen to be eating the world's best sports diet, and know that you are, that knowledge will also have the same effect. Trust in Mother Nature's best bounty—the nutrients abounding in wholesome foods. You'll always win with good nutrition!

For additional readings on this topic, see Appendix B.

SECTION III

Weight Control

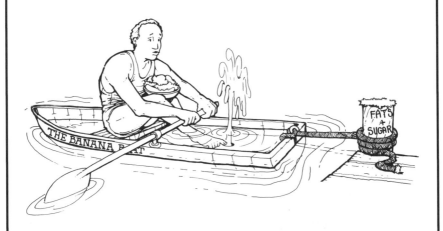

CHAPTER 13

A Matter of Fat

Many athletes hate their body fat with a vengeance. One of my clients, a collegiate swimmer, grabbed her inner thigh and exclaimed with disgust, "See this? I hate it. I can't seem to lose this handful of flab no matter how hard I train or how many leg lifts I do." A basketball player yanked a handful of flesh around his hips and cringed. "This spare tire drives me crazy. I hate the way it bulges over my uniform's shorts. I always feel so fat compared to my teammates."

Mind you, neither of these athletes was overweight or overfat. Compared to the average American, they were trim and well below normal fat levels. The swimmer was 19 percent fat; the average woman is 25 percent fat. The basketball player was 10 percent fat; the average man is about 15 percent fat.

However, when they compared themselves to their teammates, they perceived themselves as blimps. Like most scantily clad athletes, they somehow always seemed to be too fat and were never able to get "perfectly" thin. Even among the nation's top women runners—a very lean group of women—body fatness is an issue. When surveyed about their desired weight, more than half wanted to lose about 2 to 4 pounds (Clark, 1988).

Although excess body fat is simply excess baggage that slows us down, we do need a certain amount of fat for our bodies to function normally. Fat, or adipose tissue, is an *essential* part of our nerves, spinal cord, brain, and cell membranes. Internal fat pads the kidneys and other organs; external fat offers a layer of protection against cold weather. For the "reference" man, essential fat comprises about 3 to 5 percent of body weight (that is, 4-1/2 to 7-1/2 fat pounds for a 150-pound man). In comparison, the "reference" woman has about 12 percent essential fat (15 fat pounds for a 125-pound woman). Table 13.1 further describes the various levels of body fatness.

Table 13.1   Body Fat Standards

Classification	Image	% Fat	
		Males	Females
Very low fat	skinny	7–10	14–17
Low fat	trim	10–13	17–20
Average fat	normal	13–17	20–27
Above normal fat	plump	17–25	27–31
Very high fat	fat	25+	31+
Essential fat	—	3–5	11–13

Note. Data from *Being Fit: A Personal Guide* by B. Getchell and W. Anderson, 1982, New York: John Wiley & Sons. Copyright © 1982. Adapted by permission.

Women store essential fat in their hips, thighs, and breasts. This is readily available to nourish a healthy infant should a woman become pregnant. The handful of fat that the swimmer grabbed on her inner thigh included essential fat that Mother Nature wanted her to have. No wonder she had trouble losing that small bulge; it was supposed to be there.

Body-Fat Facts

We're all familiar with the "fats of life"—the fat thighs, tummy bulges, and spare tires. Here's a short trivia quiz to test your fat knowledge.

1.   **True or False**: To spot-reduce the fat around the stomach and hips, you should incorporate sit-ups into your exercise program.

False. Spot-reducing sounds like a great idea, and entrepreneurs have made fortunes by designing exotic exercise machines that "melt away" fat spots if not overnight, then at least within a week. According to exercise physiologist Frank Katch at the University of Massachusetts at Amherst, the concept of spot-reducing is hokum (Katch, 1984). That is, you can't reduce through vigorous exercise only the fat cells in one localized area of your body. The fat burned during prolonged exercise comes from all areas of the body, not just from the part of the body being worked most vigorously; and it is the burning of fat, and not muscle movement in itself, that reduces body fat.

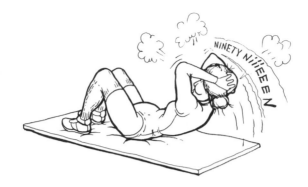

Katch commandeered 19 college students to do 5,004 sit-ups over the course of 27 days. He compared fat measurements from the exercised and unexercised parts of their bodies and found them to be equivalent at the beginning and end of the study. Both abdominal and shoulder-blade fat experienced similar changes. Granted, the stomach muscles got stronger, but the stomach fat changed at the same rate as the other body fat. Efforts to spot reduce just didn't work!

To lose fat, you have to eat fewer calories than you burn off. That way, you'll dip into the energy reserves stored in that spare tire and flatten it down a bit. Exercise can help you to burn off those calories, but you'll lose the fat everywhere, not just in one place.

2.   True or False: If you become injured and are unable to exercise for a week, your muscles will turn into fat.

False. Muscle does not turn into fat nor does fat turn into muscle. They are two separate entities and not interchangeable. Perhaps you've noticed a fat layer on roast beef or pork chops. A similar fat layer occurs with humans. The fat tissue is a layer of fat-filled cells that covers the muscles. Muscle is the protein-rich tissue that performs exercise. When you exercise, you build up muscle tissue. When you consume fewer calories than you expend, you reduce the fat layer.

If, due to injury or illness, you are unable to exercise, your muscles may lose their tone, but they won't turn into fat. Unexercised muscle tissue actually shrinks in size. For example, Joe, a skier, broke his leg and was shocked to see how scrawny his calf looked when the cast was removed 5 weeks later. Once Joe started exercising again, he rebuilt the muscle to its original size.

If you overeat (as often happens with inactive athletes who are also bored, depressed, and hopeful that chocolate chip cookies will cure all ailments), you will become fatter. I often counsel wounded football players who gain 10 to 20 pounds after an injury. They continue to eat lumberjack portions although they need fewer calories. The extra fat takes up more space than the muscle, and the players feel and look flabby.

3. True or False: Cellulite is a special kind of fat that appears after a person has yo-yo'd on and off several diets.

False. Cellulite is a fad description of the bulging "orange peel" appearance of fat that sometimes appears on the hips, thighs, and buttocks. Although much is written about cellulite, little is actually understood about it. Some medical professionals believe that the bumpy, waffle-like appearance of cellulite may result from restrictions of connective tissue separating fat cells into compartments. If you overeat and fill the fat cells, the compartmental restrictions may cause the fat to bulge.

Women are afflicted by cellulite more than men because their skin is thinner and their fat compartments are larger and more rounded. Also, women tend to deposit fat in their hips, thighs, and buttocks—areas where cellulite appears easily—and men tend to deposit fat around their waists.

Some medical specialists suspect a genetic predisposition toward cellulite may exist. If a mother has cellulite, the daughter is likely to suffer the same affliction. Cellulite generally appears as a person ages because the skin loses its elasticity and becomes thinner.

Body Image: Waiting for the Right Body

Mary, a short and stocky skier, was sensitive about her bulky body. Friends had teasingly referred to her as a fire hydrant. As I measured her body fat, Mary anxiously awaited the moment of truth.

"Your weight is fine, Mary," I said. "You simply have a lot of muscle and big bone structure. You have very little excess fat." Although Mary perceived herself as being overweight, she was actually quite lean and not overfat.

Visual appearance and body weight are deceptive for athletes who mistakenly tend to compare themselves to their teammates. We all come in different sizes and shapes, most of which is genetically determined. Although you can change your body to a certain extent by losing or gaining weight, you can't do a complete make-over. You can lose the excess baggage, but sometimes you just can't convert those thick thighs into toothpicks. One of my clients, Janice, complained, "I just hate my 'mega-legs.' Can't I do anything to slim them down?"

I questioned Janice about her mother's, sisters', aunts', and grandmothers' legs. She acknowledged, "We all have thunder thighs. They're the trademark of our family." I invited Janice to reevaluate her body shape goals and become a bit more realistic in her expectations given this genetic predisposition. ''You may not like your legs, Janice, but they're yours forever. You can trim them a bit by losing some fat, but you're unlikely to transform them into toothpicks. I recommend that you let go of your anger, accept yourself for who you are—a sincere and caring person—and focus on the things in life that really matter. You're wasting a lot of mental energy worrying about your thighs. Enjoy your life instead of putting life on hold as you wait for the right body.''

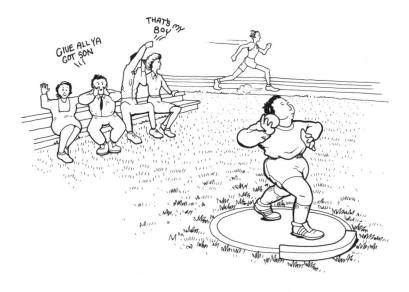

Janice is just one of many of my clients who express deep frustration about their body images. Unfortunately, the media promotes a clear message that everyone is supposed to look like a celery stalk, and that the pears and apples among us are overweight gluttons who should be ashamed of our seeming slothfulness. Far from the truth! We all come in different sizes and shapes unique to our genetic makeup; just as some of us have thick hair, others have thin hair, some have blue eyes and others have brown eyes. No one seems to care about hair thickness or eye color, but the media has made us all care about body fatness. As a result, too many self-conscious people feel inadequate because of repeated failures at transforming themselves into a shape they just aren't meant to be. For example, one husky high school soccer player wanted to transform herself into a petite ballerina, an unrealistic vision. She thought she could just diet away the excess pounds and become lean and lanky. She failed to recognize that she had little fat to lose—that most of her weight was solid muscle, not flabby fat.

Body Types

Like it or not, you're born with a specific body type that you are unable to completely overhaul! The three standard body-type classifications are these:

Ectomorph—Relatively long legs and arms, narrow fingers and toes, and a delicate bone structure.

Mesomorph—Heavy bone and muscle development; broad hands and a muscular chest.

Endomorph—Round and soft, often with slender wrists and ankles, and relatively small facial features.

Body shapes can also be classified into four categories*:

BOX   PEAR   INVERTED HOURGLASS
**   TRIANGLE**

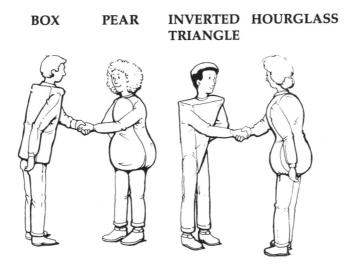

The Pear
The pear normally has narrow shoulders, a small chest, and an average waist. Fat concentration is usually in the hips and thighs.

The Box
The box often looks straight up and down, with no visible waistline. Fat concentration is often in the waist.

---

*Note. From LIFESTEPS® : Weight Management: A Summary of Current Theory and Practice, courtesy of NATIONAL DAIRY COUNCIL®.

The Inverted Triangle
Inverted triangles usually have broad shoulders and narrow hips. Fat concentration is generally in the chest.

The Hourglass Figure
Broad hips and chest, and a small waist. Fat concentration is in both the chest and hips.

Body-Fat Measurements: Fat or Fiction?

When I counsel athletes who have a poor concept of their ideal weight, I measure their body fat rather than rely on a scale and height-weight charts. The fat measurement helps put into perspective the proportion of an athlete's body that is muscle and bone, essential fat and excess fat. The scale provides a meaningless number because it doesn't indicate the composition of the pounds. Some pounds are generally desirable muscle weight, others are less desirable fat weight. Obviously, the muscle weight contributes to top athletic performance in most sports. The fat weight is the bigger concern because excess fat can slow you down.

Believe me, judging from the tension that radiates from a weight-conscious athlete's body, I believe that little in life is more anxiety-provoking than getting your body fat measured! This number unveils the real truth. Hulky football players are often humbled to learn that 20 percent of their brawn is flab—excess fat they lug around, not solid, steely muscle. Weight-conscious gymnasts are often thrilled to learn that they're trimmer than they thought.

If you want to have your body fat measured, you'll certainly want to have it done correctly by a qualified health professional using the most accurate method, and eliminate any possibility of being told that you're fatter than you really are. Inaccurate readings send people into a tizzy! If you later want to get remeasured, always try to have it done by the same person using the same technique to insure greater consistency.

The most common methods for estimating percent fat include these:

1. *Underwater weighing,* which sounds intriguing and traditionally has been considered the most accurate method.

2. *Skinfold calipers,* which are more commonplace and less sensational.

3. *Electrical impedance,* which is a snazzy, computerized method.

When it comes to measuring body fat, there's no method to date that's 100-percent accurate. Underwater weighing, calipers, and electrical impedance each have potential inaccuracies. The following information evaluates these options to help you decide the best way to estimate your ideal weight, should you want to quantify the fats of life.

Underwater Weighing

With underwater weighing, the subject exhales all the air in his or her lungs and then is weighed while submerged in a tank of water. Actually, this technique does not measure body fat. It measures *body density*. Body density translates mathematically into percentage fat. During the translation, however, significant error can creep into the picture. The equations for translating density into fat are most appropriate for "the standard male." This excludes a lot of very thin runners and very muscular body builders. Nevertheless, the same equations are inappropriately used for girls on the high school swim team, 50-year-old marathoners, and professional football players.

Children and senior citizens differ in body densities. This raises questions about the differences in densities among all types of athletes. The anorexic ballerina with osteoporotic, low-density bones is likely to get a percent-fat estimate that is far from the truth, because her body density is unlike that of the standard male.

Errors with underwater weighing also stem from the inexperience of the victim being weighed. If you've never been submerged into a weighing tank, you're likely to be nervous and may incompletely exhale all the air in your lungs before going under the water. This will affect the density reading. Exercise physiologists have estimated that as little as 2 cups of air can affect body fat measurements by as much as 3 to 5 percent. Intestinal gas can also disrupt the accuracy, as can poorly calibrated equipment. Many portable underwater weighing systems (the kinds that show up at road races, health fairs, and runners' expos) may lack the precision of a weighing system used in a research laboratory.

Needless to say, if you're looking for a 100-percent perfect measurement, underwater weighing has sources of error. But so do the other methods.

Skinfold Calipers

Skinfold calipers—large "pinchers" that measure the thickness of the fat layer at specific body sites—are best used by health professionals who have been well trained in the technique. Sports-active people often are measured by poorly trained technicians at crowded health fairs or fitness events.

A hasty measurement an inch above or below the established "pinch point," can add 5 to 15 millimeters of fat to the measurement. Those little millimeters can translate inaccurately into a high reading.

I often get phone calls from frenzied athletes who were measured at a health fair and are told that they're overfat when they suspect that they're really not that obese. When I carefully remeasure them in my unrushed, uncrowded office, I can get a much better reading. I can also use my professional judgment to determine whether the number I get seems to be reasonable for that person. The "eyeball method" is fairly reliable!

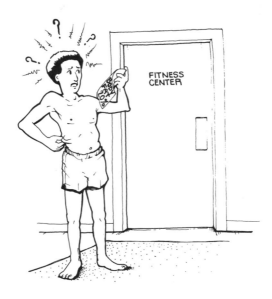

Individual fat patterns also contribute to inaccurate calculations. For example, one female skier had inherited abnormally fat arms. An arm measurement is used in many conversion formulas. According to one calculation that used this arm measurement, the skier's body was 28 percent fat, but according to another method that adjusted for the fat arms, her body was 19 percent fat. That's quite a variation.

Even accurate measurements commonly translate into erroneous information because of inappropriate conversion equations. To be most accurate, the measurements from a runner, wrestler, body builder, or gymnast should be plugged into sport-specific conversion equations. This seldom happens for the average athlete. In harried situations such as some health fairs, the technicians are unlikely to take the time to switch formulas. They can even forget to convert from male to female equations. One rushed technician incorrectly used a man's formula on a woman. The poor lady ended up with measurement of 8 percent more fat than she really had and a depressed state of mind. She had frustrations about her weight until she decided to get her fat remeasured under more peaceful conditions.

As you can now understand, the accuracy of skinfold measurements greatly depends upon the precision of the technician, the accuracy of the caliper, and the appropriateness of the conversion equations. Repeated measurements by different technicians using different calipers and different equations can yield widely different results.

Nevertheless, skinfold caliper measurements can be an excellent way to monitor changes in body composition. I often record on a monthly basis the measurements of people losing a significant amount of weight through regular exercise. By comparing the numbers (either as measurements in millimeters or converted into percent fat), the dieters can monitor changes. This use of calipers is highly precise, assuming, as I mentioned earlier, that the same technician measures the dieter each time, using the same calipers and the same conversion equations.

Bioelectrical Impedance

Bioelectrical impedance is the new kid on the block when it comes to measuring body fat. This computerized system sends an imperceivable electrical current through the body via an electrode attached to the wrists and ankles. The amount of water in the body affects the flow of the current. Because water is only in fat-free tissue, the current flow can be translated into percentage body fat. The machine is portable, easy to use, and popular at road races and health fairs.

This method, like others, also can be problematic, particularly among athletes. You'll get an inaccurate reading if you are dehydrated, so don't bother to get measured after hard exercise or after you've had any beer or alcoholic beverages. Both of these factors affect the water level in your body and will alter the reading. Other factors that may affect the accuracy of the measurement include premenstrual bloat, food in the stomach, and carbo-loaded muscles (water gets stored along with the carbohydrates). If you're improperly positioned during the test say, with part of your arms touching your body), you'll also get an inaccurate reading. This can easily happen in crowded exhibitions.

Even if you're in water balance and accurately positioned, you still might receive an incorrect measurement. The calculations are based on the assumption that the standard person is 73 percent water. However, young people tend to be 77 percent water, older folks 71 percent. Exercise scientists are developing new prediction equations to resolve this problem.

Until researchers find the definitive method, here's my advice. Consider body-fat measurement as a measurement against itself that reflects changes in your body as you lose fat, gain muscle, shape up, and slim down. Don't expect more accuracy than is possible. The standard error is plus or minus 3 percent. If you're measured at 15 percent, you might be 12 percent or 18 percent. That doesn't take into account another 3-percent biological error due to individual variations.

Your best bet is to see how the measurements change over time. Have the same person take them at bi-monthly intervals over the course of a year. Calipers are generally the most convenient, most precise, and least expensive method. They provide the information you need to assess your percent fat.

Even better than entrusting your fate to a random number, I strongly recommend that you listen to your body. Each person has a set point weight at which the body tends to hover. You may slightly overeat one day, slightly undereat the next, but your weight will stay more or less the same. If you drop below this natural weight, your body will scream at you. You may feel hungry and become obsessed with food and chronically fatigued. If you're above your set point, you'll feel fat and flabby.

My experiences counseling athletes of all ages and abilities indicate that each person really does know his or her comfortable weight zone. Tricia, a 5'2" master's swimmer, acknowledged, "I can diet down to 110 pounds—an appropriate weight for the average person of my height. But I wouldn't be able to stay there. My body is most comfortable at 117 to 120. That's heavier than most people of my height, but that's what's normal for me. I fit in with the rest of my family—everyone is heavy-set."

She had learned through years of unsuccessful dieting that she'd never be able to fit her ideal body image of being perfectly thin. She has now accepted her build and recognizes that she can healthfully participate in sports regardless of the few extra pounds.

A Weighted Issue

I advise against weighing yourself daily on a scale. The scale is your friend when it indicates that you're lighter, but it all too easily becomes the enemy when it indicates unwarranted weight gain. Paul, a marathoner, clearly remembers, "One morning I got so mad at the scale. It told me I'd gained 3 pounds and I'd been starving myself for half a week. I angrily jumped up and down on it until it broke. That's the last time I've weighed myself!" Paul can laugh now when he recalls that story, but he wasn't laughing at that time.

A scale measures not only fat but also muscle gain, water, food, intestinal contents, the glass of juice you drank just prior to being weighed, and so on. And it tells you information that may be irrelevant. For example, if you increase your exercise program, decrease

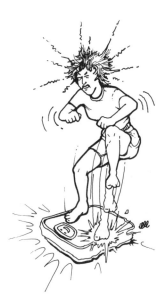

your food intake, build up muscle, and lose fat, the scale may indicate that your weight has remained the same. You'll feel thinner, look thinner, your clothes will be looser, but you may not get the psychological rewards because the scale may have dampened your spirits. Scales can also be inaccurate.

On the other hand, runners, racquetball players, and other athletes who perspire heavily often prefer to weigh themselves after a hard workout. They fool themselves with this false weight. During exercise, they may have lost 5 pounds. That's 5 pounds of sweat, not fat.

The only time to weigh yourself (if you insist) is the first thing in the morning. Get up, empty your bladder, and then step on the scale before your eat or drink anything. You'll be weighing your body, pure and simple. If you weigh yourself at the end of the day, you'll also be weighing your dinner, beverages, and other foods that are in your intestines. And be sure to keep in mind that people inherit different body types that vary in weight even if the same height. Not everyone is designed to be as thin as a fashion model nor light as a feather.

CHAPTER 14

How to Lose Weight and Maintain Energy

Most athletes believe they will always be too fat and never be too thin. Although this is far from the truth, I continue to be surprised by the number of lean athletes who openly express their fear of becoming obese and their frustrations with trying to maintain their desired low weight. They've been influenced by advertisements, cultural standards, and their peers to believe that thin is good and thinner is better. This is why body-fat measurements (see chapter 13) can be a helpful prerequisite to a weight-reduction program. By knowing their body composition and how it compares to reasonable standards, weight-conscious people can gain a realistic perspective on weight goals.

Some competitive athletes, such as wrestlers, dancers, gymnasts, figure skaters, and distance runners, strive to be extremely light and lean. Other recreational exercisers simply want to trim off the excess flab and improve their self-image. Regardless of motives for wanting to be thin, the overwhelming concern among sports-active dieters is how to lose weight and yet maintain energy for training.

High-energy, low-calorie reducing is not impossible. You can lose weight and continue to enjoy a high-energy sports diet. The trick is to wisely choose what and when you eat.

Carbohydrates for the Weight-Conscious

Like many athletes, Jan, a high school runner and constant dieter, was confused about how to lose weight during training. "I know that, for running, I'm supposed to eat carbohydrates for muscle fuel. But

186

for dieting, I'm supposed to avoid those fattening carbohydrates. How can I fuel my muscles and still lose weight?'' Like many victims of fad diets, Jan thought that carbohydrates were fattening.

As I mentioned in chapter 7, carbohydrates are not fattening. Excess fats are the true dietary demon. One teaspoon of carbohydrate has only 16 calories; that same amount of fat has 36 calories—more than twice as many. Butter, margarine, oil, mayonnaise, salad dressing, and grease are obvious fats; fats are also hidden in meat, cheese, peanut butter, nuts, and other protein foods. These highly fatty foods, and not carbohydrates, are what you should avoid.

Your body can very easily store excess dietary fat as body fat. You're more likely to burn off excess carbohydrates. If you've traded in a small carbohydrate-rich, virtually fat-free baked potato (100 calories) for a half-cup of protein- and fat-rich cottage cheese (120 calories), you've made a poor choice. The same goes for eating spoonfuls of peanut butter straight from the jar, thinking that's better for your diet than snacking on crackers. You'd be better off eating the plain potato or crackers and easily burning off their carbohydrates.

Do Low-Carbohydrate, High-Protein Diets Work?

Dieters who lose weight quickly by following high-protein, low-carbohydrate regimens are losing considerable water weight in addition to fat-weight. They eat fewer calories than usual. Instead of having eggs and buttered toast for breakfast, they have just eggs—and eat 300 fewer calories. At dinner, instead of having fish and a baked potato smothered with sour cream, they have fish alone. They believe they lose weight by eliminating the carbohydrates. In truth, they lose weight by eliminating calories.

When John, a lightweight oarsman, switched from a high-protein to a high-carbohydrate, low-fat diet, he was thrilled with his success. ''I can't believe that these carbohydrates aren't making me fat! I'm losing weight and still have energy to train.''

John had come to me the previous week feeling tired, overweight, and unsuccessful with his high-protein regimen: cottage cheese, hard boiled eggs, and broiled chicken. After explaining to John why carbohydrates are not fattening, I designed a high-carbohydrate low-fat, moderate-protein sports diet that would help him make weight yet provide sufficient energy to train. Here is that basic diet:

> *Breakfast*: cereal with low-fat milk, a banana, and juice
>
> *Lunch*: broth-type soup, a sandwich without mayonnaise or butter, and low-fat milk

Snack: fruit or low-fat yogurt

Dinner: a potato, vegetables, and a small portion of lean protein

Snack: fruit or crackers

John expressed fear of eating so much starch. I invited him to experiment with the recommendations for 1 week. He hesitatingly agreed to take my advice and follow the plan. Needless to say, he successfully lost weight.

Researchers have shown that pure carbohydrates are less fattening than pure fats. For instance, in one study by Swiss investigator Dr. Kevin Acheson, 12 subjects were monitored for a 14-hour period during which each ingested nothing but 2,000 calories of carbohydrates (sugar). Acheson measured the subjects' metabolic responses and found that only 40 of the excess carbohydrate calories were converted into body fat. The subjects' metabolic paths had shifted to preferentially burn off most of the carbohydrates; far fewer of the excess calories were converted into body fat than are converted after a standard meal in which the ingested calories include fat calories (Acheson, 1984).

In studies where subjects were fed either excess carbohydrates or excess fats, the subjects fed the high-fat diet gained more weight than the subjects fed the high-carbohydrate diet. In the Vermont Studies on the Effects of Long-term Overfeeding (Sims, 1976), the volunteers (prisoners) who ate extra portions of the standard prison diet required 7 months and about 120,000 to 180,000 excess calories to increase their body weight by 20 to 25 percent. Those who ate the basic prison diet but consumed the extra calories in fat (margarine, salad oil, and special butter cookies), gained the same amount of weight in only 3 months with only 20,000 to 40,000 excess calories. In addition, the fat overeaters easily maintained that abnormally high weight as compared to the carbohydrate overeaters, who had to eat 30 percent more calories than expected to maintain their higher weight.

Such research emphasizes the fact that carbohydrates are not fattening. Fat calories, however, do turn into body fat. The crucial factor is that fats are more fattening than carbohydrates because we convert ingested fats into body fat more efficiently than we convert carbohydrates into body fat. The metabolic cost of converting excess dietary fat into body fat is only 3 percent of the ingested calories, but the cost of converting excess carbohydrates into body fat is 23 percent (Sims, 1987). Simply stated, excess fats are more fattening than excess carbohydrates. Therefore, if you're destined to overeat and want to suffer the least weight gain, you'll be better off overindulging in raisins (carbohydrates) than in peanuts (fat).

Here's the bottom line: Delete the obviously fatty foods and enjoy the carbohydrates! As an athlete, it's essential that you fuel your muscles with these carbohydrates; they're the foundation of both a reducing diet and a sports diet.

Meal Timing: Does It Matter When You Eat?

If you tend to eat most of your calories at night because of your hectic work or training schedule, you may have wondered whether the large evening feast makes you fat. Patrick, a 25-year old triathlete and office helper, certainly had no success with dieting by day and eating by night. "I eat only an orange for breakfast because I'm not hungry after my morning run. I don't want to eat much lunch because food in my stomach can interfere with my afternoon workout. Come evening, I try to diet but generally devour whatever food I can find in my kitchen because I'm absolutely ravenous.

"Despite all my training and attempts to diet, I haven't lost weight. It seems as though I should have wasted away to nothing by now! I haven't, and I feel very discouraged. Is that because of all the nighttime eating?"

As I mentioned earlier in chapter 3, if you feast at night you may gain weight more easily than if you ate the same amount of calories earlier in the day. You can also easily overeat at night. In one study (Halberg, 1983), subjects were allowed to eat as much as they wanted but only in one meal per day. When they had their one meal at night they tended to eat 600 calories more than when they had their one meal as breakfast. It seems that if you don't eat before evening, you cultivate an enormous appetite that is hard to satisfy; you'll undoubtedly overeat and gain weight. As Patrick rationalized, "I feel as though I deserve to eat whatever I want. I've starved myself all day, I've worked hard, I'm tired, and I need a reward."

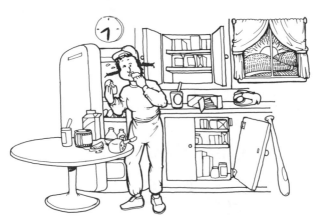

The bottom line for dieters is that you should eat during the day and be reasonable at night. You'll not only burn off the calories when you exercise and have more energy for training, but you'll also prevent yourself from getting too hungry and overeating. Remember: When you get too hungry, you may no longer have the energy to care about how much you eat. You simply want to eat . . . and eat . . .

Weight Loss Without Martyrdom

To lose weight healthfully and successfully keep it off, you should pay attention to

- *what* you eat—high-carbohydrate foods, not high-fat foods;
- *when* you eat—big breakfast, rather than big dinners; and
- *why* you eat—are you bored, stressed, lonely, or actually hungry?

These three keys can help you to implement a successful weight-reduction program that will help you to lose weight without dieting.

Actually, *diets* don't work. "Diet" is a four-letter word, and the first three letters spell D-I-E. Dieting conjures up visions of cottage cheese, grapefruit, rice cakes, and shredded wheat with skim milk. The typical dieter has very few fun memories associated with dieting. Diets teach denial and "will power." They also set the stage for going off the diet, binge eating, and developing disordered eating patterns. (In the next chapter, I'll talk more about coping with eating disorders.)

Because I'm a *dietitian*, most people assume that I put people on diets. I don't. People who go on a diet simply go off a diet. They have a 95-percent chance not only of regaining all the lost weight but also of regaining proportionately more fat than muscle. Women tend to regain that weight in their hips. After a series of yo-yo diets, one woman lamented that her body shape had changed so much that her suit size had gone from a size 14 jacket and a size 10 skirt to a size 10 jacket and a size 14 skirt. She felt frustrated, angry, and unsuccessful.

That's the sort of reason why Amy, a 39-year-old bank teller, came to me for her "last hope" diet. "I've been on every diet in the book. You name it, I've done it. I've eaten grapefruits for breakfast, lunch, and dinner. I've avoided carbohydrates like the plague. I've consumed more cottage cheese than I care to think about. I have lost at least 500 pounds—but have regained 520. Maybe *you* can put me on a successful diet?"

I explained to Amy that I wouldn't put her on a diet because diets don't work. Instead, I offered to teach her how to eat healthfully. By eating healthfully, she would lose weight. More importantly, she'd be able to exercise energetically, become and stay healthier, and learn how to keep the weight off for the rest of her life.

Successful Weight Reduction With a Dietitian

During her first meeting with me, Amy expressed her embarrassment about her inability to eat less. ''I feel childish that I can't do something as simple as lose weight. I know what I should do to lose weight, and I just don't do it.'' I assured Amy that I have helped many knowledgeable dieters who have been humbled by their lack of control over food. Successful weight reduction isn't as easy as it sounds. That's why professional advice is preferable to self-designed programs.

If you, like Amy, want to lose weight once and for all, I recommend that you get professional guidance from a registered dietitian (RD). This health professional has fulfilled specific educational requirements, has passed a registration exam, and is a recognized member of the nation's largest organization of nutrition professionals, The American Dietetic Association. Because there are no standards people have to meet to call themselves a ''nutritionist,'' you'll best protect yourself from frauds and nutrition gurus if you seek guidance from RDs.

Here are some ways to locate your local registered dietitian:
1. **Call the outpatient nutrition clinic at the community hospital.**
2. **Ask your physician for a recommendation, or inquire at a local sports medicine clinic or health club.**
3. **Call your state's dietetic association (see phone book).**
4. **Look in the yellow pages under "Dietitian" and select a name followed by "RD."**
5. **Call the American Dietetic Association (1-800-877-1600).**

Ten Tips for Successful Weight Reduction

The following steps helped Amy lose weight. They may help you develop your own winning way with food, especially if you work together with a registered dietitian. These tips are also appropriate for people who want to maintain their present weight.

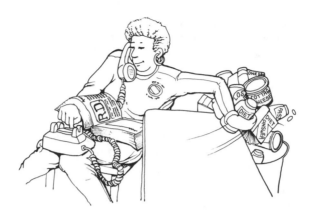

1.   Write down *what* and *when* you typically eat or drink in a day. Keep accurate food records of every morsel and drop for 3 days. Also record *why* you eat—are you stressed, hungry, or bored? Include the time and amount you exercise as well. Evaluate your patterns for potentially fattening habits such as skimping at breakfast, nibbling all day, and munching-out at night because you've gotten too hungry, or entertaining yourself with food when you're bored, or rewarding yourself with chocolate when you're stressed.

Pay careful attention to your mood when eating. Are there times when a hug and human comforting could have better nourished you than food? Eating a tub of popcorn can divert your anger, but does it resolve the problem that triggered the eating?

If you eat for reasons other than fuel, you need to recognize that food is simply fuel, nothing more, nothing less. Food becomes dan-

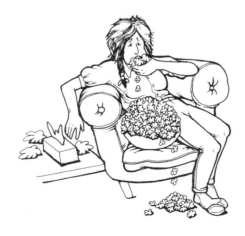

gerously fattening when it's abused for entertainment, comfort or stress reduction.

2.   Become aware of meal timing. If you're good during the day and bad at night, experiment with having a bigger breakfast and lunch, and a lighter dinner. See chapters 3 and 4 to review how eating earlier in the day prevents you from getting too hungry, losing control, and overeating in the evening.

3.   Roughly estimate the number of calories you need for normal daily activity to maintain your weight by multiplying your weight by 13 if sedentary or 15 if moderately active. You need to add more calories for significant amounts of exercise. Refer to Table 14.1 for guidelines.

You might be surprised to learn your caloric needs. Keep in mind that this number is only a rough estimate because individuals vary. This estimate assumes, for instance, that you have a normal

Table 14.1   Calories Burned During Exercise

| Exercise Category | kcal*/min of exercise | | Activities |
	Men	Women	
Light	2–5	1.5–3.5	Walking, reading a book, driving a car, shopping, bowling, fishing, golf
Moderate	5–7.5	3.5–5.5	Pleasure cycling, dancing, volleyball, badminton, calisthenics
Heavy	7.5–10.0	5.5–7.5	Ice skating, jogging, water skiing, competitive tennis
Very Heavy	10–12.5	7.5–9.5	Fencing, football, scuba diving, basketball, swimming
Unduly heavy	>12.5	>9.5	Handball, squash, cross-country skiing, paddleball, fast running

*Although we commonly refer to *calories*, the scientific measure is *kilocalories* (kcals).
Note. Data from *Nutrition, Weight Control and Exercise* (3rd ed.) by F. Katch and W. McArdle, 1988, Philadelphia: Lea and Febiger. Adapted by permission.

metabolism; which is a big assumption! Many athletes (weight-conscious athletes, in particular) are energy efficient—that is, they have adapted to needing fewer calories than the average person. You might want to add or subtract 200 to 300 calories from the total, depending on how you perceive your food requirements. A registered dietitian can offer a more professional estimate.

4.   Subtract 500 to 1,000 calories per day from your maintenance requirements to estimate the number of calories that you should eat for weight loss. I recommended that Amy knock off 300 calories of food (her evening snacks), burn off 200 more calories with aerobic exercise, and expect to lose about 1 pound per week. In comparison, a football player who has gained weight during the off-season by eating 4,500 calories a day could easily subtract 1,000 calories of food, burn off 500 to 1,000 calories with aerobic exercise, and expect to lose about 3 or 4 pounds per week.

Theoretically, if you eat 500 fewer calories than you burn off per day, you should lose 1 pound per week because 1 pound of fat is the equivalent of 3,500 calories:

$$500 \text{ cal} \times 7 \text{ days/week} = 3,500 \text{ cal/week} = 1 \text{ lb body fat}$$

Unfortunately, this is not always the case. Some people adapt to eating less, particularly those who either have dieted for many years or have no excess body fat to lose. Frustrating, but true.

Don't try to subtract more than one third of your caloric needs. If you cut back too much, you may lose muscle. Adding aerobic exercise, such as brisk walking or cross-country skiing, is preferable to subtracting food. If you don't eat enough, you'll consume too few of the nutrients that protect your health and promote top performance.

5.   Distribute your estimated caloric allotment evenly throughout the day, ensuring that you'll have energy to exercise. Plan three meals plus an afternoon or evening snack. Amy's meal pattern was this:

Breakfast:	500 cal
Lunch:	500 cal
Snack:	200 cal
Dinner:	500 cal

6.   Eat slowly! Overweight people tend to eat faster than their normal-weight counterparts. The brain needs about 20 minutes to receive the signal that you've eaten your fill. No matter how much you consume during those 20 minutes, the satiety signal doesn't move any faster. Brothy soup is an excellent first course for dieters because it takes time to eat and decreases the appetite for the main entree.

Try to pace your eating time so that you eat less and avoid the discomfort that often accompanies rapid eating.

7.   Eat your favorite foods on a regular basis. If you deny yourself permission to eat your favorite foods, you're likely to binge. However, if you give yourself permission to eat small portions of the foods you want, you'll be less likely to blow your reducing plan. If chocolate-glazed donuts are among your favorites, have one once a week. When eating this treat, do remember to chew it slowly, savor the taste, and fully enjoy it. You'll free yourself from the temptation to devour a dozen donuts in one sitting.

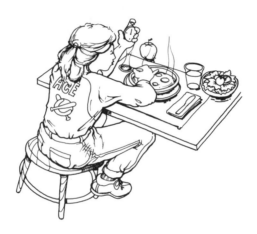

8.   Keep away from food sources that tempt you; out of sight, out of mind, and out of mouth! If you spend a lot of free time in the kitchen, you might want to relax in the den, where food is less likely to be readily available. At parties, socialize in the living room, away from the buffet table and away from the snacks. At the market, skip the aisle with the cookies and do not shop when you're hungry!

9.   Post a list of 10 nonfood activities to do (instead of eating) when you're bored, lonely, tired, or nervous. For example, you might want to call a friend, write a letter, take a bath, water the plants, listen to music by candlelight, go for a walk, take a nap, or meditate.

10.   Think "lean and fit." Every morning before you get out of bed, visualize yourself as being slimmer and trimmer. This will help you start the day with a positive attitude. If you tell yourself that you're eating healthfully and successfully losing weight, you will do so more easily. Talking positively with yourself is important for your well-being.

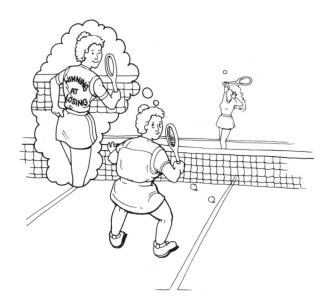

These tips helped Amy remind herself that when she ate well, she felt better and trained better. She also felt better about herself. After years of unsuccessful dieting, she liked feeling successful—perhaps even more important than feeling thinner.

CHAPTER 15

Eating Disorders

Betsy, a 16-year-old runner, says that her obsessions with food began when her high school track coach advised her to lose 5 pounds—5 pounds she didn't have in excess. She ended up losing muscle and strength.

Peter, a 40-year-old lawyer, started having cookie fixations during his struggle to attain a lower-than-ever racing weight for the Boston Marathon. His diet of 1,500 calories per day consisted of nothing for breakfast or lunch, then 30 Oreos after his run. He was just too hungry to cook a healthy dinner, so he madly devoured cookies instead then panicked that he might gain weight.

Sally, a 31-year-old compulsive swimmer, reported constant food thoughts after she had lost 20 pounds. She wanted to weigh less than 100 pounds even though 110 was a good weight that she could comfortably maintain. She'd finish one meal, and then immediately start thinking about the next because she was still hungry but afraid of overeating.

Many athletes are overwhelmed by food obsessions and eating disorders. They worry continuously about what they'll eat, when and where they'll eat, how much weight they'll gain if they simply eat a normal meal with their friends, how many hours they'll have to exercise to burn off those calories, how many meals they should skip if they overeat by a few morsels, and so on. They're consumed by the endless stream of frets revolving around food, weight, exercise, and dieting.

Eating Disorders Among Athletes

Eating disorders among sports-active people seem to be on the rise. Many coaches express concerns about some of their athletes, especially those in weight-related sports such as running, gymnastics, wrestling, and lightweight crew. Research indicates that eating disorders are widespread among college athletes:

- About one third of collegiate female athletes have some type of disordered eating pattern, be it anorexia (self-induced starvation), bulimia (binge eating, followed by self-induced vomiting), laxative abuse, excessive exercise, crash diets, or other unhealthy weight-loss practices (Rosen, 1986).
- 3 percent of almost 695 athletes in midwestern colleges met the diagnostic criteria for anorexia, and 21.5 percent met the criteria for bulimia (Burckes-Miller, 1988). (See pages 200 and 201 for these diagnostic criteria.)

Approximately half of all dieters report abnormal eating binges. Weight-conscious athletes who constantly diet to be unnaturally thin are prime candidates for disordered eating patterns.

If you're among the lucky few who effortlessly maintain their desired weight, you probably think that all this talk about food is ridiculous. However, if you're a runner, dancer, gymnast, wrestler, or other weight-conscious athlete who strives to be thinner, you may experience some degree of an obsession with food.

I estimate that about 30 percent of my patients at SportsMedicine Brookline are obsessed with food, and they represent only a minority of athletes who seek professional nutrition guidance. Most food-obsessed athletes struggle on their own, often abusing exercise as well as food. They are embarrassed that they can't seem to resolve their food imbalances. They often struggle for years before asking for help. One dancer confided that I was the first person in 15 years to whom she talked about her bulimia.

Food, for these athletes, is not fuel. It's "The Fattening Enemy" that thwarts their desire to be perfectly thin. Their goal is thinness at any price—often a price of mental anguish, physical fatigue, and impaired athletic performance. One runner failed to connect her inability to finish track workouts with her "one banana a day diet." She thought she fell asleep in classes because she had stayed up too late, not because she was underfed. Such denial!

If you are anorexic or bulimic, I recommend that you seek help from a professional counselor experienced with eating disorders, as well as nutritional guidance from a registered dietitian. Extreme eating disorders generally reflect an inability to cope with life's day-to-day stresses. For example, one of my clients, a high-level executive, smothered her stress with peppermint ice cream, hot fudge sauce, and pecans. This treat certainly diverted her attention from her problems, but it didn't resolve any of them. Afraid of gaining weight, she'd burn off

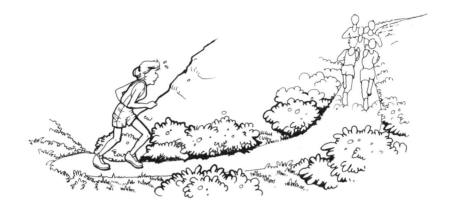

the calories with a long swim that was pure punishment. She became injured from the excessive exercise, panicked at her inability to exercise, tried to stop eating, became ravenous, binged, and then resorted to self-induced vomiting as a means to purge the calories because she could no longer swim. She came to me looking for help with food. I insisted that she also get psychological counseling to help her deal with stress.

The following case studies are typical of the clients I treat. They may sound familiar and might help those of you who constantly struggle with food and exercise.

Case Study #1: A Runner with Disordered Eating Patterns

Pete, a 42 year old runner, never was concerned about his weight until he began running 2 years ago. He felt fat compared to other runners and decided to diet. He'd grind through a 10-mile run, eat very little during the day, then devour any food in sight. "I feel so guilty about the boxes of cereal, crackers, and cookies I devour. After a binge, I won't eat dinner with my wife and children. Instead I'll go for another run to burn off the excess calories. My kids get mad at me for eating all the cookies. My wife complains that I'm neglecting the family. I'm disappointed in myself for being such a failure. I'm embarassed that I'm unable to do something as simple as lose a few pounds. I can't even eat normally now. I either diet or binge. I don't know if I should be seeing you or a psychologist."

To help Pete better balance his food and exercise goals and normalize his disordered eating patterns, I measured his percent body fat (an excellent 8 percent), determined how many calories his body required each day, and devised a meal plan to stabilize his eating. Like many of my clients, he dieted too hard for someone with little excess

---

What Is Anorexia?

The following definition is used by the American Psychiatric Association (1987):

- Intense fear of becoming obese, which does not diminish as weight loss progresses.
- Disturbance of body image; for instance, claiming to "feel fat" even when emaciated.
- Weight loss of at least 15 percent of original body weight. If under 18 years of age, weight loss from original body weight plus projected weight gain expected from growth charts may be combined to make the 15 percent.
- Refusal to maintain body weight over a minimal normal weight for age and height.
- No known physical illness that would account for the weight loss.

Note. Adapted with permission from the *Diagnostic and Statistical Manual of Mental Disorders, Third Edition, Revised.* Copyright 1987 American Psychiatric Association.

Symptoms of Anorexia: What to Look for

Significant weight loss
Hyperactivity
Compulsive exercising
Distorted body image
Intense fear of becoming fat
Loss of menstrual periods (in women)
Loss of hair
Growth of fine body hair
Extreme sensitivity to cold temperatures

Low pulse rate
Isolation from family and friends
Nervous at mealtime
Tearful, uptight, overly sensitive, restless
Spends a lot of time working or studying
Cuts food into small pieces and plays with it
Wears baggy clothing and layers of clothing

Source: Hahneman Hospital Eating Disorders Program, Boston, MA.

What Is Bulimia?

- Recurrent episodes of binge eating (rapid consumption of a large amount of food in a short period of time, usually less than 2 hours).
- At least three of the following:
  1. Consumption of high-calorie, easily ingested food during a binge.
  2. Inconspicuous eating during a binge.
  3. Termination of such eating episodes by abdominal pain, sleep, social interruption, or self-induced vomiting.
  4. Repeated attempts to lose weight by severely restrictive diets, self-induced vomiting, or use of cathartics or diuretics.
  5. Weight fluctuations greater than 10 pounds due to alternating binges and fasts.
- Awareness that the eating pattern is abnormal, and fear of not being able to stop eating voluntarily.
- Depressed mood and self-deprecating thoughts following eating binges.
- The bulimic episodes are not due to anorexia nervosa or any known physical disorder.

Note. Adapted with permission from the *Diagnostic and Statistical Manual of Mental Disorders, Third Edition, Revised.* Copyright 1987 American Psychiatric Association.

Symptoms of Bulimia: What to Look for

Frequent vomiting

Difficulty swallowing and retaining food

Swollen glands

Puffiness around face (below cheeks)

Damage to throat

Bursting blood vessels in the eyes

Loss of tooth enamel

Weakness, headaches, dizziness

Secretive behavior

Inconspicuous binge eating

Frequent weight fluctuations due to alternating binges and fasts

Overconcern with physical appearance

Petty stealing of money to buy food for binges

Source: Hahneman Hospital Eating Disorders Program, Boston, MA.

fat to lose. His weight goal was well below the set point weight he could comfortably maintain.

Pete unrealistically restricted his calories. He would run 10 miles in the morning, which expended about 1,000 calories, but he would eat nothing until lunch, when he limited himself to 450 calories. No wonder he longed for food before dinner—he was starving! I advised him to stop dieting and start eating breakfast and lunch, and to then eat reasonably at night. He changed his habits and stopped his evening binges.

Pete followed my recommendations to eat 2,600 calories divided more evenly throughout the day. "I no longer act like a maniac in front of the refrigerator, eating whatever I can get my hands on. I've decided against losing any more weight; my body just doesn't want to be thinner. I do feel great. I have energy at work. I'm less irritable. My running is improving. And most importantly, I feel in control of my food."

Case Study #2: A Triathlete with a Serious Eating Disorder

Mary, a 26-year-old advertising account executive and triathlete, had gained 8 pounds in 2 years' time despite being bulimic. She tended to overeat when work became overwhelming and she felt she couldn't do all that was expected of her. "I binge at night and then vomit. I'm exhausted from fighting with food and weight. I've stopped socializing with my friends because I'm afraid it'll present the opportunity to over-eat and that I'll be unable to purge. Instead, I spend my time training twice a day to try to lose weight. I inevitably end up at the bakery, where I buy at least six bran muffins and God only knows what else. I'm a food-aholic and just can't seem to control my intake."

Upon listening to Mary's story, I recognized that she was not only addicted to food, but also to work and exercise. She constantly pushed

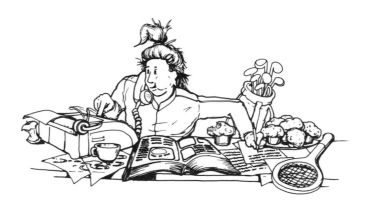

herself to meet self-imposed deadlines, weight goals, and exercise demands. She constantly felt stressed and overextended. She lacked a healthy balance to her life.

I asked if anyone in Mary's family had trouble with alcohol. She looked at me with surprise in her eyes, wondering how I guessed this family secret. Her father was an alcoholic.

At least one third of my clients with eating disorders grew up in a family with some type of dysfunction, most commonly alcohol problems. Though they themselves are not addicted to alcohol, they often express other addictive behaviors through overworking, overeating, overachieving, and overexercising. Surveys suggest that approximately one third of all children of alcoholics become bulimic (Brisman, 1984; Colins, 1985). Many disguise themselves as dedicated athletes when actually they are compulsive exercisers. The following represent traits and attitudes that researchers have identified as being characteristic of some people who grow up in an alcoholic or dysfunctional family (Wolitz, 1983):

Drive for perfection: "I'll run 120 miles per week and shed that last pound."

Desire for control: "I never touch ice cream, cookies, or white sugar, not even in a birthday cake."

Compulsive behavior: "I swim 2 miles every day, regardless of holidays, injuries, or family crises."

Mary displayed all of these traits. She had a strong drive to be perfect and a desire for control. Since childhood she had tried to be perfect to compensate for her family's problems. Now she was trying to eat the perfect diet, achieve the perfect weight, and maintain the perfect training schedule. She ran 10 miles every day, despite blizzards, illness, or fatigue (a "perfect" training schedule). She lived on calorie-free coffee and diet soda (the "perfect" diet), until ravenous hunger overwhelmed her good intentions. After she binged, she'd vomit to bring control back to her life.

I helped Mary gain a better perspective on a normal weight (by measuring her percent body fat), normal diet (by designing an appropriate meal plan), and a normal training program (by referring her to a coach). I also advised her to read some books about adult children of alcoholics, seek guidance from an appropriate counselor, and perhaps join a support group such as Al-Anon or ACOA (Adult Children of Alcoholics). For additional readings, see Appendix B.

"For years, I thought that food was the source of my struggles," she wrote in a follow-up letter. "It wasn't. Life was the problem. I'm now gentler on myself. I even let myself be imperfect. For example,

I took 3 days off from training when I went on vacation! I'm eating well and exercising healthfully, rather than pounding myself with mega-miles to burn off calories. I feel better and am at peace with myself.''

How to Help the Eating-Disordered Athlete

''I get scared when I see Alicia. She's nothing but skin and bones covered up with a baggy sweat suit. I rarely see her eat anything but sugar-free gum or lettuce topped with catsup for salad dressing. She never joins us at parties after meets because she has to study, or so she says. I think she's anorexic. What should I do?''

Deb was obviously concerned about her friend and teammate, Alicia, and was at a loss as to how to help her—if indeed Alicia was anorexic and did need help. Even health professionals can have trouble distinguishing between the ''lean and mean'' and the anorexic. Generally speaking, the athletic-anorexic exercises frantically from fear of gaining weight. In comparison, the anorexic-athlete trains hard, with hopes of improving performance. Both push themselves to perfection—to be perfectly thin or to be the perfect athlete. Often the two become intertwined.

Approximately half of all anorexics become bulimic; some purge by vomiting, others by exercising obsessively. For example, some of those long-distance runners you see exercising at all hours of the night may be purging themselves of too many calories under the guise of training.

This constant battle with food endangers an athlete's physical and mental health and overall well-being. Unfortunately, too many coaches, parents, friends, and teammates shy away from the devastating stressfulness of this self-imposed struggle for ultimate thinness. After all, how can anyone who is training and seems happy be sick?

If you suspect that your friend, training partner, child, or teammate has a problem with food, you should speak up in an appropriate manner. Anorexia and bulimia are potentially life-threatening conditions that shouldn't be overlooked. Here are 10 tips for approaching this delicate subject:

1. *Heed the signs.* You may notice that anorexics wear bulky clothes in order to hide the abnormal thinness, or that their food consumption is abnormally restrictive and spartan in comparison to the energy expended. A runner, for example, may eat only a yogurt for dinner after having completed a strenuous 10-mile workout. Perhaps you'll never see them eating in public, at home, or with friends. They find

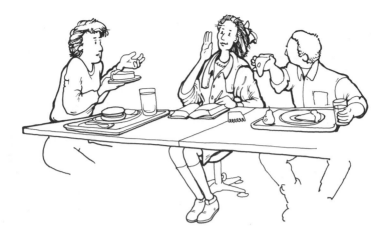

some excuse for not joining others at meals. Or if they do, they may push the food around on the plate to fool you into thinking that they're eating. You may also notice other compulsive behaviors, such as excessive studying or working.

Bulimic behavior can be more subtle. The athlete may eat a great deal of food and then rush into the bathroom. You may hear water running to cover up the sound of vomiting. The person may hide laxatives, or even speak about a magic method of eating without gaining weight. She or he may have bloodshot eyes, swollen glands, and bruised fingers (from inducing vomiting).

2. *Express your concern carefully*. Approach these individuals gently but persistently, saying that you're worried about their health. Explain that it's obvious that they have problem balancing food and exercise. Ask if they want to talk about it. Individuals who are truly anorexic or bulimic will usually deny the problem, insisting that they're perfectly fine. Share your concerns about their lack of concentration, light-headedness, or chronic fatigue. These health changes are more likely to be stepping stones for accepting help, given that the athlete undoubtedly clings to food and exercise as attempts to gain control and stability.

3. *Don't discuss weight or eating habits*. The athlete takes great pride in being perfectly thin and may dismiss your concern as jealousy. Avoid any mention of starving/binge as the issue and focus on *life* as the real issue.

4. *Suggest unhappiness as the reason for seeking help*. Point out how anxious, tired, or irritable the athlete has been lately. Emphasize that he or she doesn't have to be that way.

5. *Be supportive and listen sympathetically*. But don't expect someone to admit right away that there's a problem. Give it time, and constantly remind the athlete that you believe in him or her. This will make a difference in recovery.

6. *Offer a list of sources of professional help*. Although the athlete may deny the problem to your face, she or he may admit despair at another moment. If you don't know of local resources, ask the national organizations for the closest one (see the list at the end of this chapter).

7. *Limit your expectations*. You alone can't resolve the problem. It's more complex than food and exercise; it's a life problem. Share your concerns with others; seek help from a trusted family member, medical professional, or health service. Don't try to deal with it alone, especially if you're making no headway and the athlete is becoming more self-destructive.

8. *Recognize that you may be overreacting*. Maybe there is no eating disorder. Maybe the athlete is appropriately thin for enhanced sports performance. But how can you decide? To clarify the situation, insist upon a mental health evaluation. If necessary, make the appointment and take the athlete there yourself. Only then will you get an unbiased opinion of the degree of danger, if any. The therapist might tell you to go home and stop worrying, or might detect misery and suicidal tendencies in the athlete and encourage immediate care.

9. *Talk to someone about **your** emotions*. You may need to discuss your feelings with someone. Remember that you are not responsible for the other person's health, and you can only try to help. Your power comes from using community resources, guidance counselors, registered dietitians, members of the clergy, or eating disorder clinics.

10. *Be patient*. Recognize that the healing process can be long and arduous, but it is *always* worthwhile.

Finding Help for Eating Disorders

For more information, or for help for someone with anorexia or bulimia, contact one of these organizations:

American Anorexia/Bulimia Association
133 Cedar Lane
Teaneck, NJ 07666
(201-836-1800)

Anorexia Nervosa and Related Eating Disorders (ANRED)
PO Box 5102
Eugene, OR 97045
(503-344-1144)

Center for the Study of Anorexia and Bulimia
1 West 91 Street
New York, NY 10024
(212-595-3449)

National Anorexic Aid Society
5796 Karl Road
Columbus, OH 43229
(614-426-1133)

National Association of Anorexia Nervosa and Associated
  Disorders (ANAD)
PO Box 7
Highland Park, IL 60035

CHAPTER 16

Weight Gain
the Healthy Way

"My friends call me 'The Garbage Can,' " contended Jim, a scrawny 21-year-old collegiate athlete. "No matter how much I eat, my weight stays the same. I'll single-handedly devour a whole large pizza and then a pint of ice cream for dessert. Eating has become a chore, to say nothing of an expense. I'm tired of trying to gain weight."

Martin, a high school football player, expressed similar concerns. "I want to bulk-up before the football season and gain muscle but not fat. My coach wants me to gain 15 pounds. I've been trying all sorts of weight gain drinks—Tiger's Milk, protein powders, and amino acid pills—nothing seems to work."

When it comes to weight, most sports-active people contentedly maintain their desired weight or else struggle to lose a few pounds. Others, however, enviously wish they could add a few pounds. Many football and hockey players, body builders, and teenage boys want to gain weight by building their muscles. Some very thin and spindly athletes even wish they could gain a little fat to fill out their physique! For people struggling to gain weight, eating can be a task, food a medicine. These individuals feel self-consciously thin, hate their skinny image, and seemingly eat nonstop in hopes of putting a little "meat" on their bones. This chapter, along with chapter 11 can give you the information you need to healthfully reach your goal.

Theoretically, to gain 1 pound of body weight per week, you'd need to consume an additional 500 calories per day above your typical intake. Some people are hard-gainers and require more calories than others to add weight. For example, research subjects who theoretically should have gained 11 pounds during a month-long overfeeding study gained an average of only 6 pounds (Webb, 1983). A 9-percent increase in body-heat production partially accounted for the discrepancy, but researchers are mystified about the whole picture. What happened to the excess calories that didn't turn into fat and didn't get burned off from the higher metabolism?

In another study (Sims, 1976), 200 prisoners with no family history of obesity volunteered to be gluttons. The goal was to gain 20 to 30 pounds (20 to 25 percent above their normal weight) by deliberately overeating. For more than half a year, the prisoners ate extravagantly and exercised minimally. Yet only 20 of the 200 prisoners managed to gain the weight. Of those, only two (who had an undetected family history of obesity or diabetes) gained the weight easily. One prisoner tried for 30 weeks to add 12 pounds to his 132 pound frame, but couldn't get any fatter.

If you are a hard-gainer, take a good look at your family members. If at your age they were thin and sylphlike, you probably have inherited a genetic predisposition to thinness. You can alter your physique to a certain extent with diet and weight training, but you shouldn't expect miracles. Marathoner Bill Rodgers will never look like body builder Charles Atlas, no matter how much eating and weight lifting he does!

Most scrawny athletes believe that the best way to gain weight is to eat a high-protein diet. *False.* You don't store excess protein as muscle. The pound of steak just doesn't convert into a bigger bicep. You need extra carbohydrates, rather than extra protein, to fuel your muscles so they can do more exercise. By overloading the muscle with weight lifting and other resistance exercise, you make the muscle fibers increase in size. The exercise builds muscle, not the extra protein.

Protein powders and amino acid supplements are worthless when it comes to gaining muscle weight. They're a fruitless expense. The only reason these may work for some athletes is because the protein beverage provides additional calories. One can just as easily eat another sandwich to get those calories.

You're most likely to gain weight if you *consistently* eat larger-than-normal meals. I often counsel skinny athletes who swear they eat huge amounts of food. For example, one soccer player declared that he ate at least twice what his friends ate. However, he ate only two meals per day. Granted, he did eat a lot when he ate, but this merely compensated for the lack of breakfast and snacks.

The soccer player gained 5 pounds within 3 weeks after he started to eat three meals a day and an additional bedtime snack. ''I now look at food as my weight-gain medicine. There are times when I'm busy and tempted to skip lunch, but I remind myself that I have to take my medicine: two hefty sandwiches with two glasses of milk.''

Adam, a 6'7" high school basketball player, also chowed down on large portions. He was embarrassed whenever he'd eat with his friends because he'd eat twice what they ate. A large pizza was no challenge! When I calculated his caloric needs, he began to understand why he wasn't gaining weight. He needed about 6,000 calories per day to maintain his weight—plus more to gain weight. The pizza was 1,800. Two pizzas would have been more appropriate.

I told Adam to feed his body what it needed and stop comparing his food intake to his shorter friends. I suggested that he explain to any teasers that his body was like a limousine that needed more gas to go the distance.

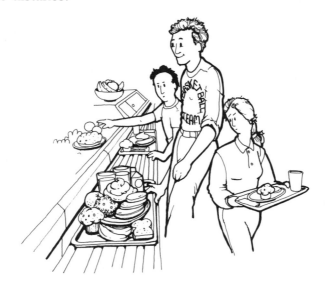

How to Boost Your Calories

To take in the extra calories you need to gain weight, you can eat

- an extra snack, such as a bedtime peanut butter sandwich with a glass of milk;
- larger-than-normal portions at meal-time; and
- higher calorie foods.

Table 16.1 offers some suggestions.

When you make your food selections, keep in mind that fats are the most concentrated form of calories. One teaspoon of fat (such as butter, oil, margarine, or mayonnaise) has 36 calories; the same amount

Table 16.1 Boost Your Calories

When food seems a medicine and every calorie counts, try boosting your intake by choosing the foods that have the most calories per serving. Small changes in your diet can make big changes in your weight.

Food	Amount	Calories
Orange juice	8 oz (1 c)	110
Cranberry juice	8 oz (1 c)	170
Bran flakes	1-1/2 c	200
Granola	1-1/2 c	780
Apple	1 lg	130
Banana	1 lg	170
Green beans	1 c	40
Corn	1 c	140
Vegetable soup	1 c	80
Split pea soup	1 c	130
Rice	1 c	190
Baked beans	1 c	260

of carbohydrate or protein has only 16 calories. Most protein foods contain fat (such as the cream in cheese, the grease in hamburgers, or the oil in peanut butter), so these foods tend to be high in calories. However, some fats, such as the saturated fat in cheese, beef, chicken skin, butter, and bacon are bad for your health. Try to limit your intake of these foods and focus on the healthful fats, such as corn oil margarine, olive oil, old-fashioned (unprocessed) peanut butter, and oily fish such as salmon and mackerel. You should still be eating the basic high-carbohydrate sports diet as described in chapter 7; you'll be adding extra unsaturated fats to that foundation.

It's a Matter of Choice

The following foods and beverages can help you healthfully boost your calorie intake:

Cold Cereal. Choose dense cereals (as opposed to flaked and puffed types), such as granola, muesli, Grape-Nuts, and Wheat Chex. Top with nuts, sunflower seeds, raisins, banana, and other fruits.

Hot Cereal.   Cooking with milk, instead of water, adds more calories and greater nutritional value. Add still more calories with mix-ins such as powdered milk, margarine, peanut butter, walnuts, sunflower seeds, wheat germ or dried fruit.

Juices.   Apple, cranberry, cranapple, grape, pineapple, and apricot have more calories than grapefruit, orange, or tomato juice. To increase the caloric value of frozen orange juice, add less water than the directions indicate.

Fruits.   Bananas, pineapples, raisins, dates, dried apricots, and other dried fruits contain more calories than watery fruits such as grapefruit, plums, and peaches.

Milk.   To boost the caloric value of milk, add 1/4 cup powdered milk to 1 cup of 2-percent milk. Or try malt powder, Ovaltine, Carnation Instant Breakfast, Nestle's Quik, and other flavorings. Mix these up by the quart to have them waiting for you in the refrigerator. You can also make blender drinks such as milk shakes, fruit smoothies, and frappés.

Toast.   Spread with generous amounts of peanut butter, margarine, and jam or honey.

Sandwiches.   Select hearty, dense breads (as opposed to fluffy types), such as sprouted wheat, honey bran, rye, and pumpernickel—the bigger and thicker sliced, the better! Spread with generous amounts of margarine or mayonnaise. Stuff with tuna salad, chicken, or other fillings. Peanut butter and jelly make an inexpensive, healthful, and high-calorie choice.

Soups.   Hearty lentil, split pea, minestrone, and barley soups have more calories than brothy chicken and beef types—unless the broth is chock full of lots of veggies and meat. To make canned soups (such as tomato or chowder) more substantial, add evaporated milk in place of water or regular milk, or add extra powdered milk. Garnish with margarine, parmesan cheese, and croutons. If you have high blood pressure, you should limit your intake of canned soups because they have a high salt content. Homemade ones are preferable.

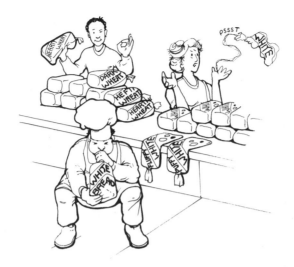

Meats.   Although beef, pork, and lamb tend to have more calories than chicken or fish, they also tend to have more saturated fat. Eat them in moderation and choose lean cuts. To boost calories, sautée chicken or fish in safflower, canola, or olive oil, or in margarine, and add wine sauces and breadcrumb toppings.

Beans, Legumes.   Lentils, split pea soup, chili with beans, limas, and dried beans are not only high in calories but also excellent sources of protein and carbohydrates.

Vegetables.   Peas, corn, carrots, winter squash, and beets have more calories than green beans, broccoli, summer squash, and other watery veggies. Add generous amount of margarine, slivered almonds, grated cheese, or sauces.

Salads.   What may start out being low-calorie lettuce can be quickly converted into a substantial meal by adding cottage cheese, garbanzo beans (chick-peas), sunflower seeds, assorted vegetables, chopped walnuts, tuna fish, lean meat, croutons, and a liberal dousing of salad dressing made with heart-healthy oils, such as olive or corn (see chapter 5).

Potatoes.   Add generous amounts of margarine and extra powdered milk to mashed potatoes. Although sour cream and gravy add significant amounts of calories, they also add saturated fats that are unhealthful for your heart.

Desserts. By selecting desserts with nutritional value, you can enjoy treats as well as nourish your body. Try oatmeal-raisin cookies, Fig Newtons, rice pudding, chocolate pudding, stewed fruit compotes, pumpkin pie, carrot cake. Blueberry muffins, corn bread with honey, banana bread, and other sweet breads can double as dessert.

Snacks. A substantial afternoon or evening snack is an excellent way to boost your calorie intake. If you don't feel hungry, just think of the food as the weight-gain medicine that you *have* to take.

Some healthful snack choices include fruit yogurt, cheese and crackers, peanuts, sunflower seeds, almonds, granola, pretzels, English muffins, bagels, bran muffins, pizza, peanut butter crackers, milk shakes, instant breakfast drinks, hot cocoa, bananas, dried fruits, and sandwiches.

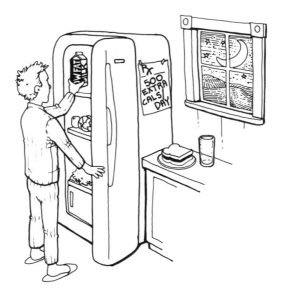

Alcohol. Moderate amounts of beer and wine can stimulate your appetite and add extra calories, particularly when consumed with snacks such as peanuts and pretzels. Because alcohol offers little nutritional value, do not substitute it for juices, milk, or other wholesome beverages. (Remember, never drink alcohol before an event; it has a dehydrating effect.)

See the sample menus in Table 16.2.

Table 16.2 5,000-Calorie Sample Weight-Gain Menus

The trick to gaining weight is to consistently eat larger-than-normal portions three times a day plus one or two snacks. These sample menus suggest healthful, high-calorie, carbohydrate-rich sports meals.

Menus	Approximate calories
Breakfast 1	
1 c orange juice	100
6 pancakes	600
1/4 c syrup	200
2 pats margarine	100
2 c low-fat milk	200
Total	1,200
Breakfast 2	
2 c pineapple juice	280
1 c granola	500
1/4 c raisins	120
2 c low-fat milk	200
1 lg banana	170
Total	1,270
Lunch 1	
4 sl hefty bread	400
1 6.5-oz can tuna	200
4 T lite mayonnaise	200
1 bowl lentil soup	250
2 c low-fat milk	200
2 oatmeal cookies	150
Total	1,400
Lunch 2	
1 7"-pita pocket	240
6 oz turkey breast	300
2 T lite mayonnaise	100
2 c apple juice	250
1 c fruit yogurt	250
1 lg muffin	300
Total	1,440
Dinner 1	
1 med cheese pizza	1,400
2 c low-fat milk	200
Total	1,600
Dinner 2	
1 breast chicken	300
2 lg potatoes	400
2 pats margarine	100

Menus	Approximate calories
1 c peas	100
2 biscuits	300
2 T honey	100
2 c low-fat milk	200
Total	1,500
Snack 1	
1 peanut butter and jelly sandwich	
2 sl hearty bread	200
3 T peanut butter	300
3 T jelly	150
Milkshake:	
1-1/2 c low-fat milk	150
1/4 c milk powder	100
2 T chocolate powder	150
Total	1,050
Snack 2	
2 bagels	400
3 oz lite cheese	260
2 c cranberry juice	340
Total	1,000

Patience is a Virtue

By taking the prescribed 500 additional calories per day, you should see some weight gain. Theoretically, you should be able to gain 1 or 2 pounds per week if you eat 500 to 1,000 additional calories per day. Be sure to include muscle-building exercise (weight workouts, push-ups) to promote muscular growth rather than just fat deposits. Consult with the trainer at your school, health club, or gym for a specific exercise program that suits your needs.

If you don't gain weight, look at your family members to see if you inherited a naturally trim physique. If everyone is thin, accept your fate and concentrate on improving your athletic skills. If you capitalize on being light, swift, and agile, you'll be able to surpass the heavier hulks that lack your speed.

Also, keep in mind that most people gain weight with age—your turn will probably come! All too often, scrawny young athletes fatten up once they get out of school and start working. For example, Wes, a 30-year-old photographer and former football player, reported with a sigh, ''I was skinny all through high school. In college, my football coach insisted that I gain weight by eating extra buttered bread, piles of french fries, and mounds of ice cream. I developed quite a liking for these foods. I continued to eat them even after I'd reached my weight-gain goals. Voilà—look at me now!!! I'm 60 pounds overweight and can barely walk, to say nothing of play football. I long for those days when I was lean and mean.''

With a low-fat nutrition program, Wes did lose weight over the course of a year. That fall, he coached an after-school football program. Needless to say, he carefully advised the thin kids to be patient, to eat healthfully, and to develop smart, lifelong eating habits.

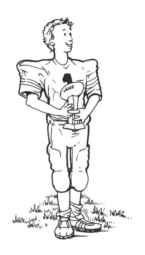

Recipes For Health and Fitness

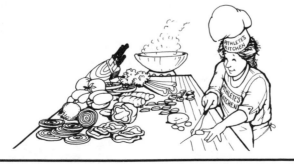

Philosophies on Food

Active people generally prefer to spend their time exercising rather than preparing meals. The following recipes are designed to help you spend minimal time preparing maximal nutrition. Even the least skilled of cooks will be able to prepare meals that taste good, invest in health and top sports performance, are quick and easy to fix, and use commonly available ingredients. These recipes appropriately fit into a low-fat, high-carbohydrate, heart-healthy sports diet. Some have moderate amounts of sodium. For those of you who require a salt-restricted diet due to high blood pressure, simply eliminate or reduce the salt or salty foods in the recipes.

Many of the recipes are tried-and-true favorites contributed by athletes or food-lovers themselves. Others are recipes I've adapted from higher-fat versions. I've tried to compile a collection of "safe" foods that will be popular with all members of the family—athletes and support crew alike. My primary criterion for selection was whether the taste-testers requested a second helping.

How To Use the Nutrition Information With the Recipes

The calorie and nutrient information provided with each recipe represents approximate values. Remember that your total daily caloric intake should be about 60 percent carbohydrates, 25 percent fat, and 15 percent protein. To convert these targets into grams, multiply your daily calorie need (see chapter 14) by the targets, and then divide the carbohydrate and protein products by 4 and the fat product by 9. For example, for an active woman who needs about 2,000 calories per day, the calculations are as follows:

60% carbohydrate x 2,000 cal = 1,200 carbohydrate cal = 300 g carbohydrate

25% fat x 2,000 cal = 500 fat cal = 55 g fat

15% protein x 2,000 cal = 300 protein cal = 75 g protein

Some of the recipes are higher in protein and fat than others, so add up your daily grams to be sure that you balance your intake. The calorie and nutrient information provided with each recipe represents approximate values.

Microwave Cooking

Unlike conventional cooking, in which food is surrounded by heat and cooks from the outside in, microwaved foods cook from the inside out. Microwaves (high-frequency energy waves similar to radar, TV, and radio waves) cook your food by causing water molecules in the food to "jiggle." This causes friction and results in heat. Hence, only items containing moisture get hot. Paper plates, glassware, and other microwave-safe materials transfer the waves without absorbing them. Aluminum foil and metal reflect the waves.

Microwave ovens are a blessing for those of us who eat on the run; today at least half of all American households have one. I highly recommend them for active folks who want to eat well and spend little time cooking and cleaning. With just a 1-day cookathon, you can have a week's worth of food ready to pop into the microwave. For example, on weekends, I might make a big pot of chili or curry or a chicken-rice casserole; I'll freeze some and leave the rest in the refrigerator, creating a ready supply of microwave entrées.

Breads and Breakfasts

Any way you slice them, breads are one of the favorite carbohydrates for active people. Here are some baking tips to help you prepare the yummiest of breads.

1. The secret to light and fluffy quick breads, muffins, and scones is to stir the flour lightly and only for 20 seconds. Ignore the lumps! If you beat the batter too much, the gluten (protein) in the flour will toughen the dough.

2. Breads made entirely with whole wheat flour tend to be heavy. In general, half whole wheat and half white flour is an appropriate combination. Many of these recipes have been developed using this ratio. You can alter the ratio as you like. When substituting whole wheat for white flour in other recipes, use 3/4 cup whole wheat for 1 cup white flour.

Breads made with 100-percent whole wheat flour do offer more nutritional value than those made with white flour. However, if you or your family dislikes whole wheat products, compensate by consistently eating wholesome bran cereals, fruits, and vegetables. These will replace the nutrients lost in the refining process. You needn't feel obligated to limit your intake to only 100-percent whole wheat breads.

3. These recipes have reduced sugar content. To reduce the sugar content of your own recipes, use one third to one half less sugar than indicated; the finished product will be just fine. If you want to replace white sugar with honey, brown sugar, or molasses, use only 1/2 teaspoon baking powder per 2 cups flour and add 1/2 teaspoon baking soda. This prevents an "off" taste.

4. Most quick bread recipes instruct you to sift together the baking powder and flour. This method produces the lightest breads and best results. In some of these recipes, I direct you to mix the baking powder in with the wet ingredients and gently add the flour last. My method is easier, produces an acceptable product, and saves time and energy.

5. To prevent breads from sticking, either use nonstick baking pans or place a piece of waxed paper in the baking pan before pouring the batter. For me, waxed paper works best. After the bread has baked, I let it cool for 5 minutes, tip it out of the pan, then peel off the paper.

6. To hasten cooking time, bake quick breads in a 8″ × 8″ square pan instead of a loaf pan. They will bake in half the time. You can also bake muffins in a loaf or square pan, eliminating the hard-to-wash muffin tins!

Breads
Applesauce Raisin Bread
Banana Bread
Beer Bread
Irish Soda Bread
Moist Corn Bread
Orange-Oatmeal Bread
Three-Seed Yeast Bread
Whole Wheat Raisin Quick Bread
Cinnamon Oat Bran Muffins
Honey Bran Muffins
Griddle Scones

See also: Tortilla Crisps.

Breakfasts
Granola
Oat Bran Deluxe
Oatmeal Pancakes

See also: French Toast With Cheese, Fruit Smoothie, Crunchy Peanut Butter Sandwich, Maple Graham Shake, and suggestions in chapter 3.

Applesauce Raisin Bread

Yield
16 slices

This moist bread can double as a dessert.

1 16-ounce jar applesauce (1 1/2 cups)
1 egg or 2 egg whites
1/2 – 3/4 cup sugar
1/4 cup oil, preferably safflower or canola
2 teaspoons cinnamon

1 teaspoon salt
1 teaspoon baking powder
1 teaspoon baking soda
1 cup raisins
1 1/2 cups flour, half whole wheat and half white

1. Preheat the oven to 350°.
2. Combine the applesauce, egg, sugar, oil, cinnamon, salt, baking powder, and baking soda. Mix well. Add the raisins.
3. Gently mix in the flour. Stir 20 seconds or until just moistened.
4. Pour into a lightly oiled or wax-papered 4" × 8" loaf pan. Bake for 45 minutes or until a toothpick inserted near the middle comes out clean.
5. Let cool for 5 minutes before removing from the pan.

Nutrition Information

145 calories per slice; 2,300 calories per recipe
One slice: 25g (70%) carbohydrate, 2g (5%) protein, 4g (25%) fat

Banana Bread

Yield
12 slices

For best results, use well-ripened bananas.

3 large well-ripened bananas

1 egg or 2 egg whites

2 tablespoons oil, preferably safflower or canola

1/3 cup milk

1/3 – 1/2 cup sugar

1 teaspoon salt

1 teaspoon baking soda

1/2 teaspoon baking powder

1 1/2 cups flour, half whole wheat and half white

1. Preheat the oven to 350°.
2. Mash the bananas with a fork.
3. Add the egg, oil, milk, sugar, salt, baking soda, and baking powder. Beat well.
4. Gently blend the flour into the banana mixture and stir for 20 seconds or until moistened.
5. Pour into a lightly oiled or wax-papered 4" × 8" loaf pan.
6. Bake for 45 minutes or until a toothpick inserted near the middle comes out clean.
7. Let cool for 5 minutes before taking out of the pan.

Nutrition Information

140 calories per slice; 1,600 calories per recipe
One slice: 24g (70%) carbohydrate, 3g (10%) protein, 3g (20%) fat

Beer Bread

A dinner bread with wonderful yeasty aroma that goes well with soups and stews.

3 cups flour, half whole wheat and half white

1 1/2 tablespoons baking powder

1 1/2 teaspoons salt

2 tablespoons sugar

1 egg or 2 egg whites, slightly beaten

2 tablespoons oil, preferably safflower or canola

1 12-ounce can beer

1. Preheat the oven to 350°.
2. Combine the flour, baking powder, salt, and sugar. Mix well.
3. In a small bowl, beat together the egg and oil; add the beer. Add to the flour mixture, stirring gently until just blended. Do not overbeat or the bread will be tough.
4. Pour into a lightly oiled or wax-papered 4" × 8" loaf pan. Bake for 50 to 55 minutes or until a toothpick inserted near the middle comes out clean.
5. Let cool for 5 minutes before removing from the pan.

Nutrition Information

140 calories per slice; 1,700 calories per recipe
One slice: 25g (70%) carbohydrate, 7g (20%) protein, 1g (10%) fat

Irish Soda Bread

This bread's distinctive flavor comes from the caraway seeds, which add sweetness without sugar. For variety, bake this into muffins.

2 cups flour, half whole wheat and half white

2 teaspoons baking powder

1/2 teaspoon baking soda

1/2 teaspoon salt

2 teaspoons caraway seeds

1 cup raisins

1 egg

1/3 cup oil, preferably safflower or canola

1 cup low-fat milk

1. Preheat the oven to 375°.
2. In a mixing bowl, combine the flour, baking powder, baking soda, salt, and caraway seeds. Mix in the raisins.
3. Beat together the egg, oil, and milk; add to the flour mixture. Gently stir just until blended.
4. Put the dough into an oiled or wax-papered 9" round cake pan, forming it into a round loaf.
5. Bake for 35 to 40 minutes or until nicely browned.
6. Slice into wedges.

Nutrition Information

165 calories per wedge; 2,000 calories per recipe
One slice: 23g (55%) carbohydrate, 2g (5%) protein, 7g (40%) fat

Moist Corn Bread

Yield
9 squares

The cream-style corn in this bread makes the final product very moist, unlike the many corn breads that are dry and crumble easily. When made with the cheese and/or beans, it becomes a hearty lunch.

1 cup yellow cornmeal

2 teaspoons baking powder

1/2 teaspoon salt

1 egg or 2 egg whites

3/4 cup low-fat milk

1/4 cup oil, preferably safflower or canola

1 16-ounce can cream-style corn

Optional: 1 tablespoon chili powder; 4 ounces shredded cheddar cheese, preferably low-fat; 1 cup kidney or pinto beans.

1. Preheat the oven to 350°.
2. In a medium bowl, combine the cornmeal, baking powder, and salt (and chili powder, if desired).
3. Optional: Sprinkle cheese and beans onto the cornmeal mixture and gently mix in.
4. Beat together the egg, milk, oil, and cream-style corn. Add to the cornmeal mixture; stir just until blended. Do not overbeat.

5. Pour into an oiled or wax-papered 8″ x 8″ baking pan. Bake about 40 minutes, or until golden and a toothpick inserted near the center comes out clean. Let stand for 10 minutes before cutting into squares.

Nutrition Information

180 calories per square; 1,620 calories per recipe
One slice: 25g (55%) carbohydrate, 5g (10%) protein, 7g (35%) fat

Orange-Oatmeal Bread

Yield
12 slices

Nice for breakfast or snacks. Spread with orange marmalade for a special treat.

1 egg or 2 egg whites	**1/2 cup orange juice**
1/4 cup honey	**1 1/2 cups uncooked rolled oats**
1/4 – 1/3 cup oil, preferably safflower or canola	**1 1/2 teaspoons baking powder**
	1 teaspoon salt
1/2 cup low-fat milk	**1 1/2 cups whole wheat flour**

Optional: 1 tablespoon grated orange rind; dash nutmeg; 1/2 cup chopped almonds; 1/2 cup raisins; 1/2 cup chopped apricots.

1. Preheat the oven to 400°.
2. Beat together the egg, honey, oil, milk, and orange juice.
3. Stir in the oats and let stand for 1 or 2 minutes. Add grated orange rind, if desired.
4. Add the baking powder, salt, and flour. Mix just until blended. Do not overbeat.
5. Pour the batter into a lightly oiled or wax-papered 4″ × 8″ loaf pan.
6. Bake for 45 to 55 minutes or until nicely browned.

Nutrition Information

170 calories per slice; 2,050 calories per recipe
One slice: 25g (60%) carbohydrate, 4g (10%) protein, 5g (30%) fat

Three-Seed Yeast Bread

Yield
16 slices

This bread is delightfully chock-full of goodies and tastes delicious, especially toasted. Try adding raisins or other dried fruit in place of the seeds.

1 tablespoon yeast	**2 teaspoons salt, as desired**
1 1/2 cups warm water	**1/2 cup sesame seeds**
1/2 cup molasses	**1/2 cup poppy seeds**
1/2 cup oil, preferably safflower or canola	**1/2 cup sunflower seeds**
2 1/2 cups raw bran (not cereal-type)	**3 1/2 cups whole wheat flour**

1. Mix the yeast, warm water, and molasses; let stand for 5 minutes.
2. Add the oil, raw bran, salt, seeds, and 2 1/2 cups whole wheat flour. Mix well, then turn out onto floured surface; knead in the rest of the flour until the dough is smooth and elastic—about 10 minutes. You might need more or less flour, depending on the particular brand.
3. Place the dough in a lightly oiled bowl, cover with plastic wrap, and let rise in a warm place for about an hour or until doubled. To shorten preparation time, omit this step and let bread rise once, in the pan, before baking.
4. Punch the dough down, shape it into a loaf, and put it into a lightly oiled 4" × 8" loaf pan. Cover and let rise again until almost doubled.
5. Bake at 350° for about 55 minutes, or until it sounds hollow when tipped out of the pan and tapped on the bottom with your fingers.

Nutrition Information

240 calories per slice; 3,800 calories per recipe
One slice: 30g (50%) carbohydrate, 6g (10%) protein, 10g (40%) fat

Whole Wheat Raisin Quick Bread

This makes a large loaf—enough for breakfast and yummy peanut butter sandwiches for lunch!

1 1/2 cups low-fat milk	1 teaspoon salt
2 tablespoons vinegar	1 1/2 teaspoons baking powder
1/2 cup molasses	1 1/2 teaspoons baking soda
1/2 cup sugar	1/2 cup white flour
1/4 cup oil	2 1/2 cups whole wheat flour
1/2 cup raisins	

1. Preheat the oven to 350°.
2. In a bowl, make soured milk by mixing the milk and vinegar. Let stand 5 to 10 minutes.
3. Mix together the remaining ingredients, except for the flour. Beat well.
4. Gently add the flour, stirring until just blended.
5. Pour into a lightly oiled or wax-papered 4" × 8" loaf pan.
6. Bake for 50 to 60 minutes, or until a toothpick inserted near the center comes out clean.

Nutrition Information

185 calories per slice; 3,000 calories per recipe
One slice: 32g (75%) carbohydrates, 5g (10%) protein, 4g (20%) fat

Cinnamon Oat Bran Muffins

These muffins are a tasty way to boost your oat bran intake. I often add chopped apples, pears, peaches, or other fruits to the batter for variety.

1 1/2 cups oat bran, uncooked	2 tablespoons oil, preferably safflower or canola
1/4 cup brown sugar	
1 teaspoon cinnamon	1 3/4 cup low-fat milk
1 teaspoon salt, as desired	1 cup flour, half whole wheat and half white
2 teaspoons baking powder	
1 egg or 2 egg whites	

Optional: 1 cup chopped fruit (apples, peaches, pears, etc.); 1/2 cup chopped nuts; 1/2 cup raisins or chopped dried fruit.

---

1. Preheat the oven to 400°. Line muffin tins with paper baking cups or use nonstick pans.
2. In a medium bowl, combine the oat bran, brown sugar, cinnamon, salt, and baking powder. Mix well.
3. Beat the egg with the oil; add the milk, then combine with the oat bran mixture. Gently blend in the flour, mixing until just moistened.
4. Fill the muffin cups 2/3 full. Bake about 20 minutes or until a light golden brown.

Nutrition Information

130 calories per muffin; 1,550 calories per recipe
One muffin: 20g (60%) carbohydrate, 5g (15%) protein, 4g (25%) fat

Honey Bran Muffins

Yield
12 muffins

Bakery muffins are often made with more fat and less bran than is optimal for health. These muffins are a super alternative.

1/2 cup low-fat milk mixed with 1 teaspoon vinegar (or 1/2 cup buttermilk)

1 1/2 cups All-Bran cereal

1 cup hot water

1/3 cup honey

1/4 cup oil, preferably safflower or canola

1/2 teaspoon salt

1 egg or 2 egg whites, beaten

1 teaspoon baking soda

1 1/2 cups flour, half whole wheat and half white

Optional: 1/2 cup raisins; 1/2 cup chopped nuts; 2 tablespoons poppy or sunflower seeds.

---

1. Preheat the oven to 400°. Line muffin tins with paper baking cups (or use nonstick muffin pans).
2. Make buttermilk by mixing the milk and vinegar. Let stand for 5 to 10 minutes.
3. Combine the bran cereal, hot water, honey, oil, salt, and egg. Let stand for 1 or 2 minutes.

4. Add the buttermilk, then the flour with the baking soda stirred into it. Mix gently until just blended. Do not overbeat!

5. Fill the muffin cups 2/3 full.

6. Bake for 20 to 25 minutes or until a toothpick inserted near the center comes out clean.

Nutrition Information

160 calories per muffin, 1,900 calories per recipe
One muffin: 26g (65%) carbohydrate, 2g (5%) protein, 5g (30%) fat

Griddle Scones

Yield
10 scones

These look like plump pancakes, but they are eaten like biscuits— especially tasty with strawberry jam! I generally make them on top of the stove, but you can also bake them in the oven at 425° for about 20 minutes.

1 cup low-fat milk mixed with 2 teaspoons vinegar

2 cups flour, half whole wheat and half white

2 tablespoons sugar

2 teaspoons baking powder

1/2 teaspoon baking soda

1/2 teaspoon salt

1/4 cup oil, preferably safflower or canola

Optional: 1/2 cup raisins, currants, blueberries, or other fruit; 1/2 teaspoon cinnamon.

1. Combine the milk and vinegar and set aside for 10 minutes.

2. In a medium bowl, mix together the flour, sugar, baking powder, baking soda, and salt.

3. Add the milk and oil. Gently stir to make a soft dough.

4. Heat a nonstick griddle (or lightly oiled skillet) over medium heat. Drop in the dough by tablespoons; pat into biscuit shape.

5. Cover and let brown on one side for about 4 minutes. Flip, partially cover, and brown on the other side. (Don't pat them with the spatula or they'll end up heavy and flat rather than light and fluffy!)

6. Wrap the scones in a clean towel to keep them warm.

Nutrition Information

150 calories per scone; 1,500 calories per recipe
One scone: 20g (55%) carbohydrate, 4g (10%) protein, 6g (35%) fat

Granola

Store-bought granolas are often prepared with coconut oil or another highly saturated fat. By making your own, you can use a heart-healthier oil— and less of it. Add extra dried fruits, rather than nuts and sunflower seeds, to boost the carbohydrate value.

4 cups rolled oats, old-fashioned or quick

1/4 cup oil, preferably safflower or canola

1/4 – 1/2 cup brown sugar, maple syrup, or honey

1/4 cup water

Optional: 1 teaspoon vanilla; 1 or 2 teaspoons cinnamon; 1 cup raisins, chopped dates, dried apricots, apple, or other dried fruit; 1/2 cup sunflower and/or sesame seeds; 1/2 cup wheat germ; 1/2 cup millet and/or kasha; 1/2 cup chopped almonds, cashews, or walnuts.

1. Preheat the oven to 300°.
2. In a large bowl, combine the oats and sugar (and cinnamon, if you like). Combine the oil and water (and vanilla, if desired); mix well with the oats.
3. Spread in a large baking pan.
4. Bake for 10 minutes, stir to toast evenly, then bake 10 minutes more.
5. While the mixture is still hot, stir in optional ingredients, as desired. Let cool.
6. Store in an airtight container.

Nutrition Information

200 calories per 1/2 cup; 2,000 calories per recipe
1/2 cup: 28g (55%) carbohydrate, 5g (10%) protein, 8g (35%) fat

Oat Bran Deluxe

Oat bran is a favorite snack before my morning run. It not only settles well but also helps to lower blood cholesterol. The following suggestions add variety to oat bran breakfasts.

2/3 cup oat bran

1/4 teaspoon salt, as desired

2 cups water (or low-fat milk)

Your choice of mix-ins:

Fruits: fresh or dried apple, banana, pineapple, raisins, dates, apricots, applesauce; canned fruit.

Nuts and seeds: chopped almonds, walnuts, sunflower seeds, sesame seeds, peanut butter.

Flavorings: cinnamon, vanilla, maple syrup, honey, molasses, jam, brown sugar, or even garlic powder!

---

1. Cook the oat bran according to package directions (making a double serving so that you'll have adequate calories for a "sports breakfast").
2. To add calcium and protein, cook the cereal in milk, fortify it with extra powdered milk, top it with yogurt, and/or serve it with milk.
3. For a substantial meal that will stick to your ribs, add mix-ins that contain protein or healthful fat, such as milk, nuts, and peanut butter.

Nutrition Information

285 calories for plain oat bran (2/3 cup uncooked) with 1/2 cup low-fat milk
One serving: 44g (60%) carbohydrates, 17g (25%) protein, 5g (15%) fat

Oatmeal Pancakes

Yield
12 pancakes

For best results, let the batter stand for 5 minutes before cooking.

**1 cup flour, half whole wheat
and half white**

**1/2 cup uncooked oats (quick or
old-fashioned)**

1 teaspoon baking powder

1/2 teaspoon salt

1 cup low-fat milk

1 egg or 2 egg whites, beaten

**2 tablespoons oil, preferably safflower
or canola**

Optional: 1 tablespoon sugar.

---

1. Combine the flour, oats, baking powder, and salt.
2. Add the milk, egg, and oil. Stir until just moistened.
3. Let the batter stand while you heat a lightly oiled or nonstick griddle over medium-high heat (375° for an electric frying pan).
4. For each pancake, pour about 1/4 cup batter onto the griddle.

5. Turn when the tops are covered with bubbles and the edges look cooked. Turn only once.

6. Serve with syrup, honey, applesauce, yogurt, or other topping of your choice.

Nutrition Information

85 calories per pancake; 1,000 calories per recipe
One pancake: 13g (60%) carbohydrate, 3g (15%) protein, 3g (35%) fat

Pasta, Rice, and Potatoes

Carbohydrate-rich meals are the key to a high-energy sports diet. The following recipes can help you fuel your muscles for training and competing. A cooking tip for pasta, rice, or noodles is to add 1 teaspoon oil to the cooking water. This prevents the finished product from sticking together.

Pasta
Pasta and Veggies With Cheese
Pasta Salad Parmesan
Pasta With Pesto Sauce
Sesame Pasta With Broccoli
Spicy Chinese Noodles
Stuffed Shells

See also: Hamburger-Noodle Feast, Easy Cheesy Noodles.

Rice
Cinnamon Raisin Rice
Company Rice Salad
Honey Nut Rice
Low-Fat Fried Rice
Orange Rice

See also: Chicken and Rice With Plum Sauce, Orange Chicken, and Sweet 'N' Spicy Orange Beef.

Potatoes
Greek Stuffed Potato
Irish Tacos
Meal-In-One Potato
Mighty Mashed Potatoes

See also: Egg-Stuffed Baked Potato, Potato Snacks.

Pasta With Veggies and Cheese

Yield
4 servings

Simple as can be! Any leftovers are excellent for tomorrow's lunch, warm or cold.

8 ounces dry pasta

1 cup part-skim ricotta cheese

4 cups vegetables of your choice, such as broccoli, fresh tomatoes, mushrooms, sliced carrots, green pepper, etc.

Seasonings as desired: garlic powder, salt, pepper, oregano, parsley, basil, parmesan cheese.

---

1. Cook the pasta according to the directions on the package. Drain.
2. While the pasta is cooking, steam the vegetables until tender-crisp.
3. Mix the ricotta with the cooked pasta; add the cooked vegetables and seasonings.

Nutrition Information

350 calories per serving; 1,400 calories per recipe
One serving: 57g (65%) carbohydrate, 17g (20%) protein, 6g (15%) fat

Pasta Salad Parmesan

Yield
4 servings

The parmesan cheese adds a light "bite" to this colorful salad.

8 ounces dry pasta, preferably shells, spirals, or elbows

2 cups broccoli flowerettes or peas, steamed

2 tablespoons olive oil

1/2 cup parmesan cheese

2 cups cherry tomatoes, halved

Seasonings as desired: 1/2 teaspoon basil, 1/4 teaspoon garlic powder, 1/2 teaspoon salt, pepper.

Optional: 2 scallions, sliced, or 1/2 medium onion, chopped; red or green peppers, diced; 2 tablespoons poppy seeds.

1. Cook the pasta according to the directions on the package. Drain.
2. While the pasta cooks, steam the broccoli; chop the scallions or onion (optional).
3. Combine the cooked pasta, broccoli, (scallions), olive oil, basil, garlic powder, and salt. Mix well. Sprinkle on the cheese and toss again.
4. Chill. Add tomatoes before serving.

Nutrition Information

360 calories per serving; 1,450 calories per recipe
One serving: 54g (60%) carbohydrate, 13g (15%) protein, 10g (25%) fat

Pasta With Pesto Sauce

Yield
4 servings

In restaurants, pesto can be a deceptively high-fat meal. This recipe uses less oil, so it's better for carbo-loading but still not as high in carbohydrates as you might think.

8 ounces dry pasta

1 cup loosely packed basil leaves (or 1 box frozen chopped spinach, cooked)

1/4 cup (1 ounce) walnuts

1/4 cup parmesan cheese, grated

1 1/2 tablespoons oil, preferably olive

1–2 cloves garlic or 1/8 teaspoon garlic powder

Salt and pepper as desired

1. Cook the pasta according to package directions.
2. In a blender, combine the basil (or spinach), walnuts, cheese, oil, garlic, and seasonings. Cover and blend until smooth.
3. Combine with the cooked pasta. Serve either hot or cold.

Nutrition Information

350 calories per serving; 1,400 calories per recipe
One serving: 48g (55%) carbohydrate, 13g (15%) protein, 11g (30%) fat

Sesame Pasta With Broccoli

Yield
4 servings

Sesame paste (tahini) is the secret ingredient in this recipe. Look for tahini in the ethnic food section of the supermarket or at the health food store. If you can't find it, substitute peanut butter diluted with 1 or 2 tablespoons boiling water.

8 ounces dry pasta

2 cups fresh or frozen broccoli, chopped

1/4 cup tahini (sesame butter)

Optional: cayenne pepper, garlic powder; vegetables of your choice, such as celery or scallions.

1. Cook the pasta according to the directions on the package. Drain.
2. While the pasta is cooking, steam the broccoli until tender-crisp.
3. Add tahini to the drained pasta and mix well. Add the cooked broccoli—and the water in which it was cooked if the pasta is ''dry.'' Add vegetables (optional).
4. If desired, add a dash of cayenne pepper or garlic powder.

Nutrition Information

325 calories per serving; 1,300 calories per recipe
One serving: 50g (60%) carbohydrate, 12g (15%) protein, 9g (25%) fat

Spicy Chinese Noodles

Yield
4 servings

If you were to call this Peanut Butter Pasta, folks might groan. Call it Spicy Chinese Noodles, and they'll come back for seconds! When serving this to guests, be sure that no one is allergic to nuts—this dish can fool even the most cautious eaters.

8 ounces dry pasta

1/3 cup peanut butter, preferably chunky

3 tablespoons soy sauce

3 tablespoons vinegar

1 tablespoon sugar, as desired

1 or 2 dashes of cayenne pepper, as desired

Optional: lightly steamed green pepper strips, snow peas, chopped scallions; garlic powder.

1. Cook the pasta according to the directions on the package. Drain.
2. While the pasta is cooking, combine in a small saucepan the peanut butter, soy sauce, vinegar, sugar, and cayenne.
3. Mix together the pasta and the peanut butter sauce. Add vegetables as desired. If the pasta is "dry," add a little water to thin the sauce.

Nutrition Information

375 calories per serving; 1,500 calories per recipe
One serving: 50g (55%) carbohydrate, 15g (15%) protein, 12g (30%) fat

Stuffed Shells

Yield
4 servings

This recipe works well with either spinach or chopped broccoli. The nutmeg adds a nicely different flavor—a change from the traditional Italian seasonings.

6 ounces large pasta shells (1/2 box)	**1 tablespoon flour**
1 10-ounce box frozen chopped spinach (or broccoli)	**2 tablespoons grated parmesan**
	1/4 teaspoon nutmeg
8 ounces part-skim ricotta cheese	**1 cup spaghetti sauce**

Optional: 1/4 teaspoon oregano, salt, pepper, or garlic powder.

1. Cook the shells according to the directions on the box. Drain.
2. Steam the spinach until tender; drain well.
3. To the drained spinach, add the ricotta, flour, parmesan, and nutmeg; add oregano, garlic, salt, and pepper as desired. Mix well.
4. Stuff each cooked shell with about 1 tablespoon of the ricotta-spinach mixture.
5. Put the stuffed shells in a 9" × 9" baking pan with a little tomato sauce on the bottom. Spoon the rest of the tomato sauce over the shells.
6. Cover and bake 25 minutes at 350°.

Nutrition Information

325 calories per serving; 1,300 calories per recipe
One serving: 45g (55%) carbohydrate, 16g (20%) protein, 9g (25%) fat

Cinnamon Raisin Rice

Yield
4 servings

This goes nicely with chicken, fish, and especially Mexican bean dishes.

1 cup uncooked rice, brown or white   **1/2 cup raisins**

2 cups water   **1 teaspoon salt, as desired**

1–2 teaspoons cinnamon

1. In a saucepan, combine the rice, water, cinnamon, raisins, and salt.
2. Bring to a boil, cover, and cook over medium-low heat for 20 to 25 minutes for white rice, 45 to 50 minutes for brown rice. Add more water if needed.

Nutrition Information

160 calories per serving; 650 calories per recipe
One serving: 38g (95%) carbohydrate, less than 1g (5%) protein, trace of fat

Company Rice Salad

Yield
4 servings

Water chestnuts and artichoke hearts can easily spiff up plain rice and make it into a special treat. Although this is designed to be a cold salad, it can be served warm.

2 1/2 cups water   **1 7-ounce can sliced water chestnuts**

1 cup uncooked rice, brown or white   **1 6-ounce jar marinated artichoke**

1 teaspoon salt, as desired   **hearts**

1. Bring water to a boil. Add rice; add salt as desired. Stir.
2. Cook covered until tender: 20 to 25 minutes for white rice and 45 to 50 minutes for brown rice. Add more water if needed.
3. Gently mix in water chestnuts and marinated artichoke hearts (including marinade).
4. Chill.

Nutrition Information

160 calories per serving; 640 calories per recipe
One serving: 28g (70%) carbohydrate, 4g (10%) protein, 4g (20%) fat

Honey Nut Rice

The honey adds a touch of sweetness; the nuts, a bit of crunch.

2 cups water

1 cup uncooked rice, brown or white

1 tablespoon honey

1 teaspoon salt, as desired

1/4 cup chopped walnuts or almonds

Optional: 1/2 cup golden raisins or chopped apricots.

---

1. Bring the water to a boil.
2. Add the rice, honey, and salt. Stir.
3. Cover and cook over low heat until tender: 20 to 25 minutes for white rice and 45 to 50 minutes for brown rice. Add more water if needed.
4. Add nuts and raisins (optional).

Nutrition Information

170 calories per serving; 680 calories per recipe
One serving: 30g (70%) carbohydrate, 2g (5%) protein, 5g (25%) fat

Low-Fat Fried Rice

This is a low-fat version of what you might get in a Chinese restaurant. Use your imagination and add whatever vegetables or protein-rich foods are handy.

1 tablespoon oil

2 scallions with greens, chopped (or 1 small onion)

1 cup sliced mushrooms

1 egg or 2 egg whites, as desired

2 cups cooked rice (about 2/3 cup uncooked)

1 tablespoon soy sauce

Optional vegetables: broccoli, celery, peas, snow peas, bok choy, chinese cabbage, water chestnuts.

Optional protein: shrimp, beef, chicken, ground turkey, tofu, nuts, sesame seeds.

Optional seasonings: garlic, sesame oil, cayenne pepper.

1. Heat the oil in a large skillet or wok over medium-high heat.
2. Add scallions and mushrooms (and other vegetables and proteins, as desired); stir-fry 2 or 3 minutes.
3. Push the vegetables aside. Pour the egg into the skillet and scramble it.
4. Stir in the rice, gently separating the grains. Add the soy sauce; stir thoroughly until heated.

Nutrition Information

340 calories per serving; 680 calories per recipe
One serving: 30g (60%) carbohydrate, 9g (10%) protein, 10g (30%) fat

Orange Rice

Yield
4 servings

This goes nicely with chicken, pork, or fish dishes.

1 1/2 cups water   **1 cup uncooked rice, brown or white**
1/2 cup orange juice

Optional: 1 teaspoon salt or 2 chicken bouillon cubes; 1 teaspoon sugar, dash of nutmeg, or dash of cloves.

1. Bring the water, juice, and salt or bouillon (if desired) to a boil.
2. Add the rice and optional seasonings; stir. Cover and cook over low heat until tender: 20 to 25 minutes for white rice and 45 to 50 minutes for brown rice. Add more water if needed.

Nutrition Information

115 calories per serving; 460 calories per recipe
One serving: 26g (90%) carbohydrate, 2g (10%) protein, trace of fat

Greek Stuffed Potato

Yield
2 servings

While you're at it, make extra for tomorrow's lunch or dinner—if these last that long!

2 large baking potatoes, 8 ounces each   **1 10-ounce box frozen chopped spinach, thawed and squeezed dry**

2 ounces feta cheese, crumbled

Optional: 2 tablespoons parmesan cheese; salt, pepper, garlic powder.

---

1. Bake the potatoes at 425° for 45 to 60 minutes.
2. When the potatoes are done, scoop out their meat into a small bowl, being careful not to burn your fingers!
3. Add the spinach, cheeses, and seasonings to your taste. Mix.
4. Fill the potato skin with the mixture and bake 10 minutes longer to blend flavors.

Nutrition Information

260 calories per serving; 520 calories per recipe
One serving: 39g (60%) carbohydrate, 13g (20%) protein, 6g (20%) fat

Irish Tacos

Yield
2 servings

These potatoes will make you say "O' lé!"

2 large baking potatoes, 8 ounces each

1/2 15-ounce can pinto beans

1/2 cup chili sauce

2 ounces shredded cheddar cheese, preferably low-fat

Optional toppings: chopped scallions, tomatoes, lettuce; salsa.

---

1. Bake the potatoes at 425° for 45 to 60 minutes, or "zap" them in the microwave oven about 6 to 8 minutes, and let them stand for 1 or 2 minutes.
2. Heat the beans with the chili sauce.
3. Split the cooked potatoes and puff them up. Spoon on the beans with chili sauce; top with the cheese.

Nutrition Information

400 calories per serving; 800 calories per recipe
One serving: 70g (70%) carbohydrate, 25g (25%) protein, 2g (5%) fat

Meal-in-One Potato

Yield
1 serving

Baked potatoes are a particularly convenient food for those who exercise before dinner. If the potato bakes while you work out, it will be ready when you are!

1 large baking potato   **2/3 cup low-fat cottage cheese**

Optional seasonings: scallions, onions; Italian seasonings, garlic powder; crumbled blue cheese, parmesan cheese.

———————————————

1. Bake the potato at 425° for 45 to 60 minutes.
2. Slit it open by cutting an X on top, and puff it up.
3. Spoon on cottage cheese mixed with seasonings of your choice.

Nutrition Information

275 calories per serving
One serving: 38g (55%) carbohydrates, 24g (35%) protein, 3g (10%) fat

Mighty Mashed Potatoes

Yield
1 serving

This dish is "mighty" because it's fortified with protein and calcium from powdered milk. It's also rich in fiber, made with potato skins to save time and nutrients. For more protein, add a scoop of cottage cheese.

1 large (8-ounce) potato with peel,   **1/3 cup milk powder**
  diced   **Salt and pepper as desired**
1/2 cup water

Optional: chopped onion; cottage cheese, low-fat cheese; mashed tofu.

———————————————

1. Cook the potato in the water in a covered pan about 15 to 20 minutes, or until tender when pierced with a fork. Do *not* drain the cooking water.
2. With a potato masher or big spoon, mash together the potato and the cooking water.
3. Add the milk powder and seasonings as desired.

Nutrition Information

225 calories per serving
One serving: 44g (80%) carbohydrate, 12g (20%) protein, trace of fat

Vegetables

Vegetables are perfectly delicious when served plain, without added flavorings. The trick is to cook them until tender-crisp and still flavorful. Limp, overcooked veggies can lose their appeal as well as some of their nutrients.

In general, vegetables contain negligible amounts of protein and fat but are packed with carbohydrates.

The first 5 recipes offer basic advice about cooking methods. Nutrition information is provided only for the final 2 recipes. Tables 1.4 and 7.4 (*Comparing Vegetables, Carbohydrate Content of Commonly Eaten Foods*) provide more nutrition information.

Recipes
Baked Vegetables

Chinese Vegetables: An Introduction

Microwaved Vegetables

Steamed Vegetables

Stir-Fried Vegetables

Carrots in Orange Juice

Stir-Fried Broccoli With Sesame Seeds

See also: Pasta With Pesto, Pasta With Veggies and Cheese, Stuffed Shells, Sesame Pasta With Broccoli, Egg-Drop Soup, Fish and Broccoli Soup, Low-Fat Fried Rice, and Greek Stuffed Potato.

Baked Vegetables

If you're baking potatoes, chicken, or a casserole, you might as well make good use of the oven and bake the vegetables, too! Wrap them in foil to save yourself clean up time.

To bake vegetables:

1. Either wrap the vegetables in foil or put them in a covered baking dish (with a small amount of water). Some popular combina-

tions include eggplant halves sprinkled with garlic powder; zucchini or summer squash halves covered with onion slices; carrot chunks; sweet potato slices and apples.

2. Bake at 350° for 20 to 30 minutes (depending on the size of the chunks) until tender-crisp.

3. When you open the foil, be careful about escaping steam so that you don't get burned.

Chinese Vegetables: An Introduction

If you're bored by the same old veggies—broccoli, green beans, carrots, corn, and peas—be adventurous! Try some of the Chinese vegetables found at larger grocery stores or Chinese markets. They tend to have a mild, inoffensive flavor that even picky eaters enjoy.

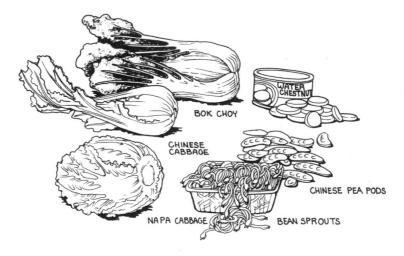

My favorites include these:

Bok choy. Slender white stalks with dark green, leafy tops. Bok choy is sweet and mild-tasting, good either raw or cooked. Simply cut off the root end, separate the stalks, and slice diagonally. Cut leaves into 1'' strips. Stir-fry, steam, or add to soups or vegetable dishes.

Chinese cabbage. Flat, white ribs with pale, cabbage-colored leaves. This has a mild flavor and can be nicely stir-fried, steamed, or added to soups, salads, or vegetable dishes.

Napa. A light cabbage-colored vegetable that comes in a bunch like celery but has broad stalks with crinkled leaves. It has a mild, sweet flavor and is good stir-fried or in salads, soups, or vegetable dishes.

Chinese pea pods. The flat, green pods are deliciously sweet and crunchy. Eat the whole pod! Rinse in water, trim the stems, and enjoy them raw in salads, as a snack, or in stir-fry dishes.

Bean sprouts. These crunchy little strands are a fun addition to stir-fried dishes, salads, soups, and casseroles. Raw or cooked, they have a mild flavor and a nice crunch.

Water chestnuts. Canned, sliced water chestnuts are a crunchy addition to stir-fry dishes, salads, or entrées. They're also a low-calorie snack alternative to munching on celery stalks!

To prepare any of these Chinese vegetables:

- Stir-fry them according to the recipe for Stir-Fried Vegetables (next page).
- Add them to chicken broth and enjoy them in the form of Chinese vegetable soup.
- Eat them raw in salads.

These vegetables blend well with the recipes for Low-Fat Fried Rice, Egg Drop Soup, Fish and Broccoli Soup, and Scallops Baked in Foil.

Microwaved Vegetables

Microwave cookery is ideal for vegetables because it cooks them quickly and without water, thereby retaining a greater percentage of nutrients than with conventional methods.

To microwave vegetables:

1. Wash the vegetables and cut them into bite-size pieces. Put them on a plate and cover them with plastic wrap. If the pieces vary in thickness, arrange them in a ring with the thicker portions towards the outside of the dish.

Optional: Sprinkle with herbs (basil, parsley, oregano, garlic powder), soy sauce, or whatever suits your taste.

2. Microwave until tender-crisp. The amount of time will vary according to your particular oven and the amount of vegetable you are cooking. You'll learn by trial and error. Start off with 3 minutes for a single serving; larger quantities take longer. Remember, the vegetables will continue cooking after they're removed from the oven, so plan that into the time allotment.

Steamed Vegetables

Here are some basic guidelines for steaming vegetables:

1. Wash the vegetables thoroughly to remove soil. Cut into the desired size.
2. Put 1/2 inch of water in the bottom of a pan with a tight lid. Bring to a boil, then add the vegetables. Cover tightly; or, put the vegetables in a steamer basket, and put this into a saucepan with 1 inch of water (or enough to prevent the water from boiling away). Cover tightly and bring to a boil.
3. Cook over medium heat until tender-crisp—generally 5 to 10 minutes.
4. Drain the vegetables, reserving the cooking liquid for soup or sauces—or even for drinking as vegetable broth.

Optional: Sprinkle vegetables with herbs before or after cooking. I generally add basil and oregano to zucchini squash, ginger to carrots, and garlic powder to green beans. Be creative!

Stir-Fried Vegetables

Vegetables stir-fried until tender-crisp are very flavorful, but they do have more fat than steamed vegetables. If you're watching your weight, be sure to add the least possible amount of oil.

Safflower and canola oils are among the heart-healthiest choices for stir-frying. For a wonderful flavor, add a little sesame oil (available in the Chinese or natural food section of larger supermarkets or health food stores).

Although a wok is popular for stir-frying, any large skillet or saucepan can do the job. I prefer a cast-iron frying pan.

To stir-fry vegetables:

1. Wash, drain well (to prevent oil from spattering when the vegetables are added) and cut the vegetables of your choice into bite-sized pieces or 1/8-inch slices. Whenever possible, slice vegetables diagonally to increase the surface area; this allows faster cooking. Try to make the pieces uniform so they will cook evenly.

Popular vegetable stir-fry combinations:
- Carrots, broccoli, and mushrooms
- Onions, green peppers, zucchini, and tomatoes
- Chinese cabbage and water chestnuts

Optional: minced garlic and/or sliced ginger root heated in the oil; 1 or 2 teaspoons soy sauce added at the end; 2 teaspoons cornstarch mixed into 1 tablespoon water to thicken the juices.

2. Heat the wok, skillet, or large frying pan over high heat. Add 1 to 3 teaspoons of safflower, canola, and/or sesame oil—just enough to coat the bottom of the pan.

Optional: Add a slice of ginger root or minced garlic to the oil; stir-fry for a minute to flavor the oil.

3. Add the vegetables that take longest to cook (carrots, cauliflower, broccoli); a few minutes later, add the remaining ones (mushrooms, bean sprouts, cabbage, spinach). Constantly lift and turn the pieces to coat them with oil. Add a little bit of water (1/4 to 1/2 cup) and cover and steam the vegetables. Adjust the heat to prevent scorching.

4. Don't overcrowd the pan. Cook small batches at a time. The goal is to cook the vegetables until they are tender but still crunchy—about 2 to 5 minutes.

Optional add-ins: soy sauce, stir-fried beef, chicken, ground turkey, tofu, or other protein of your choice to make this into a main course.

5. Thicken the juices (as they do in Chinese restaurants) by stirring in a mixture of 2 teaspoons cornstarch and 1 tablespoon water. Add more water or broth if this makes the sauce too thick.

Optional: Garnish with toasted sesame seeds or toasted nuts (almonds, cashews, peanuts); mandarin orange sections or pineapple chunks.

Carrots in Orange Juice

Yield
3 servings

This recipe is suitable for either the stove top or the oven. This combination of carrots with a hint of orange flavor goes nicely with chicken and fish.

1 pound carrots, sliced on the   **1/2 cup orange juice**
diagonal into 1/3-inch thick ovals

Optional: dash of ginger, cloves, and/or nutmeg; 1 teaspoon honey.

---

1. Put carrots in a small saucepan or casserole with a tight cover. (You might want to first peel the carrots if you're concerned about the appearance of the final product. When cooked, the peels have a slightly darker, wrinkled look.)
2. Add the orange juice and seasonings, as desired. Cover and either simmer on top of the stove about 20 minutes or bake in the oven with the rest of the meal for about 1/2 hour.

Nutrition Information

75 calories per serving; 225 calories per recipe
One serving: 17g (90%) carbohydrate, 2g (10%) protein, trace of fat

Stir-Fried Broccoli With Sesame Seeds

Yield
2 servings

This goes particularly well with broiled chicken or fish. Note: *Cooking with the oil and sesame seeds adds about 130 calories. Weight watchers might want to stick to plain steamed vegetables!*

2 stalks (1 pound) fresh broccoli   **2–4 tablespoons water**

2 teaspoons oil, preferably safflower,   **1–2 tablespoons sesame seeds**
canola, and/or sesame   **Salt and pepper as desired**

---

1. Wash the broccoli, separate the flowerettes from the stems, and cut the flowerettes into bite-size pieces.
2. Strip off the tough outer layer of the stems with a sharp knife. Slice the peeled stem into diagonal pieces.

3. Heat the oil in a heavy skillet or wok. Add the stems and stir-fry for 2 minutes. Add the flowerettes, stir, and then add the water. Cover and steam for 2 to 4 minutes or until tender-crisp.

5. Sprinkle with sesame seeds, salt, and pepper as desired.

Nutrition Information

135 calories per serving; 270 calories per recipe
One serving: 12g (35%) carbohydrate, 7g (20%) protein, 7g (45%) fat

Chicken and Turkey

The white and dark meat of chicken and turkey are excellent examples of muscle physiology. They represent two different types of muscle fibers:

• The white breast meat is primarily fast-twitch muscle fibers. These are used for bursts of energy. Among athletes, gymnasts and basketball players tend to have a high percentage of fast-twitch fibers.

• The dark meat in the legs and wings is primarily slow-twitch muscle fibers that function best for endurance exercise. Marathoners and long-distance cyclists tend to have a high percentage of slow-twitch fibers.

The dark meat (endurance muscle fibers) of poultry contains more fat than the white meat (sprint fibers) because the fat provides energy for greater endurance, so the dark meat also has slightly more fat calories than light meat:

Chicken breast, white meat: 115 calories per 4 ounces (raw)

Chicken thigh, dark meat: 130 calories per 4 ounces (raw)

The dark meat also has significantly more iron, zinc, B vitamins, and other nutrients. I recommend that non–beef eaters select dark meat poultry to boost their intake of these important nutrients.

The skin of chicken or turkey is fat-ladened. To reduce temptation, remove the skin prior to cooking.

Chicken
Baked Chicken With Mustard

Basic Steamed Chicken

Chicken and Rice With Plum Sauce

Chicken in Dijon Sauce

Chicken 'N' Cheese

Chicken Stir-Fry With Apples and Curry

Honey-Baked Chicken

Orange Chicken

See also: Mexican Baked Chicken With Beans, Stir-Fried Vegetables, and Sweet and Sour Tofu.

Turkey
Roast Turkey
Turkey Burgers

See also: Tortilla Roll-Ups, Eggplant-Tofu Parmesan, Tortilla Lasagna, Chili, Sloppy Joefus, and Low-Fat Fried Rice.

Baked Chicken With Mustard

Yield
1 serving

You can't cook chicken much simpler than this and still have it taste good enough for a special dinner. This recipe also works well with fish.

1 6-ounce piece chicken, skinned   **2 teaspoons grated parmesan cheese**
1–2 teaspoons prepared mustard

1. Line a baking pan with aluminum foil for easier cleanup. Place the chicken in the pan.
2. Brush chicken with mustard; sprinkle with parmesan cheese.
3. Bake uncovered at 350° for 20 to 30 minutes.

Nutrition Information

190 calories per serving
One serving: trace of carbohydrate, 26g (55%) protein, 10g (45%) fat

Basic Steamed Chicken

Yield
1 serving

This basic recipe lends itself to 101 creative touches.

Water   **1 6-ounce piece chicken, skinned**

1. Put 1/2 inch of water in a saucepan.
2. Add the chicken, cover tightly, and bring just to a boil. Turn down heat.
3. Gently simmer over medium-low heat for 20 to 25 minutes or until juices run clear when the chicken is poked with a fork.

Variations: Replace water with orange juice, white wine, stewed tomatoes; add seasonings (chicken bouillon cube, soy sauce, curry, basil, or thyme); cook rice along with the chicken (add extra water); make stuffing with chicken broth and stuffing mix.

Nutrition Information

165 calories per serving
One serving: trace of carbohydrate, 25g (60%) protein, 7g (40%) fat

Chicken and Rice With Plum Sauce

Yield
4 servings

Chinese plum sauce (sometimes called "duck sauce") is available in the ethnic food section of the supermarket. It has a sweet taste that deliciously complements chicken and rice.

1 1/2 cups water

1/2 cup Chinese duck sauce

1 teaspoon salt or 2 teaspoons soy sauce, as desired

1 cup uncooked rice, brown or white

4 6-ounce pieces chicken, skinned

---

1. In a medium-size covered pot, bring the water to a boil. Add the duck sauce, salt, and rice; return to a boil. If you're using brown rice, add it to the water and cook it for 20 minutes before adding the chicken.
2. Add the skinless chicken pieces. Cover and simmer over medium-low heat for 20 to 25 minutes, or until both rice and chicken are cooked. Add more water if needed.
3. Serve with a green vegetable, such as peas or spinach. If you like, add the vegetable to the cooking pot in the last 5 minutes— you'll save yourself a dish to wash!

Nutrition Information

350 calories per serving, 1,500 calories per recipe
One serving: 55g (55%) carbohydrate, 26g (30%) protein, 5g (15%) fat

Chicken in Dijon Sauce

Yield
4 servings

Delightfully different, this is my favorite "company chicken" recipe. It goes nicely with rice and carrots.

4 chicken breasts, skinned

1 cup water

2 chicken bouillon cubes

2 tablespoons Dijon-style (spicy) mustard

1/2 cup white wine (optional)

2 tablespoons flour

1/2 cup evaporated skim milk (or low-fat milk)

1. In a large saucepan, put chicken, water, bouillon, mustard, and wine (optional).
2. Cover and bring to a boil; simmer over medium-low heat for 20 minutes or until juices run clear when the chicken is poked with a fork.
3. Mix the flour with the milk.
4. Skim off any fat on top of the broth. Thicken the broth into a nice sauce by slowly stirring in the flour and milk mixture.
5. Cover and cook over low heat for 5 minutes to allow the flavors to blend.

Nutrition Information

200 calories per serving; 800 calories per recipe
One serving: 7g (15%) carbohydrate, 28g (55%) protein, 7g (30%) fat

Chicken 'N' Cheese

Yield
1 serving

To make this into a chicken cordon bleu, add a slice of lean ham along with the cheese. To make a complete dinner, bake the chicken in a covered pan with 1 1/2 cups of water and 1 cup of rice per 4 pieces of chicken.

1 6-ounce boneless chicken breast, skin removed

1/2 ounce string (mozzarella) cheese

1. Roll the chicken around the string cheese. Secure with toothpicks.
2. Bake uncovered at 350° for 25 minutes.

Nutrition Information

200 calories per serving
One serving: trace of carbohydrate, 28g (55%) protein, 10g (45%) fat

Chicken Stir-Fry
With Apples and Curry

Yield
3 servings

For curry lovers, this dinner is easy to prepare and goes nicely with rice.

**1 tablespoon oil, preferably safflower
   or canola**

1/2 cup celery, sliced on the diagonal

1 green pepper, sliced into strips

2 apples, diced

**1 pound boneless chicken breasts,
   skinned and cut into 1-inch pieces**

1 teaspoon curry

Optional: 1/4 teaspoon cumin; 1 teaspoon ground cloves; salt and pepper as desired; 1/3 cup raisins: 1/2 cup pineapple chunks.

1. Heat the oil in a large skillet or wok. Stir-fry the celery, peppers, and apples 3 to 5 minutes or until tender-crisp. Keep covered, stirring every half minute. Remove onto a platter.
2. To the skillet add the chicken; stir-fry 2 or 3 minutes, adding a little more oil if needed.
3. Add the vegetables and apples back into the skillet. Sprinkle with curry and seasonings as desired. Serve over rice.

Nutrition Information

250 calories per serving; 750 calories per recipe
One serving: 9g (15%) carbohydrate, 22g (35%) protein, 14g (50%) fat

Honey-Baked Chicken

Yield
1 serving

When you're tired of plain baked chicken, this offers a nice flavor change.

1 6-ounce piece chicken, skinned

2 teaspoons honey

1/4 teaspoon curry powder

1. Place the chicken in a baking pan. (Line the pan with aluminum foil for easier cleanup.)
2. Coat the chicken with a thin layer of honey.
3. Sprinkle with curry powder.
4. Bake uncovered at 350° for 20 to 30 minutes.

Nutrition Information

200 calories per serving
One serving: 3g (5%) carbohydrate, 25g (55%) protein, 9g (40%) fat

Orange Chicken

Yield
4 servings

This is one variation of Steamed Chicken. I sometimes add another cup of water and cook rice along with the chicken.

4 pieces chicken, skinned

1 cup orange juice

1 tablespoon cornstarch mixed in 2 tablespoons water

Optional: 1/4 teaspoon cinnamon or ginger; 1 tablespoon honey or brown sugar; salt or chicken bouillon cube, as desired; pepper.

1. Put the chicken and orange juice in a saucepan. Add seasonings as desired.
2. Cover, bring to a boil, and then simmer over medium-low heat for 20 minutes.
3. Skim the fat from the broth; thicken the broth by stirring in the cornstarch and water mixture until the broth is the desired consistency.

Nutrition Information

200 calories per serving; 800 calories per recipe
One serving: 7g (15%) carbohydrate, 25g (55%) protein, 5g (30%) fat

Roast Turkey

When I know I have a busy week ahead of me, I'll roast a turkey on Sunday so there will be plenty of food for quick sandwiches or simple dinners. Although roasting a turkey may seem a monumental task, it's really very simple, whether the turkey is stuffed or unstuffed. The oven does all the work. You simply enjoy the aromas—and then the leftovers!

The general rule of thumb for buying turkey is to allow 3/4 pound per person if the turkey weighs less than 12 pounds and 1/2 to 3/4 pound per person if the turkey weighs more than 12 pounds.

To roast a turkey:

1. Rinse the turkey inside and out under running water. Remove and discard any separable fat from around and under the skin near the body cavity.

Optional: Prepare stuffing mix according to package directions, except eliminate or reduce the butter. Stuff into the turkey cavity.

2. Fold the flap of neck skin up and over the top of the back and fasten it with either a skewer or a large safety pin.
3. Tie the legs together with string over the body opening.
4. Place the turkey on a rack (if you have one) in a shallow roasting pan.
5. Cover the turkey with a tent of aluminum foil and place in a preheated 325° oven.

Cooking times for whole turkey, unstuffed (add 5 minutes per pound if stuffed):

Pounds	Cooking time (approximate)
Less than 15 pounds	15 to 20 minutes per pound
More than 15 pounds	13 to 15 minutes per pound

To determine doneness, poke turkey with fork—juices should run clear; a meat thermometer should register 180°. If the drumsticks easily move back and forth—it's overdone! Plan an extra 15 or 20 minutes into the cooking schedule to allow the turkey to "rest" before being carved; it will slice more easily.

Nutrition Information

180 calories per serving (4 ounces cooked breast meat)
One serving: trace of carbohydrate, 36g (80%) protein, 4g (20%) fat

Optional: Low-Fat Gravy   Yield: 2 cups
1. After the turkey has cooked, pour off the grease from the roasting pan.
2. Add 2 cups water to the roasting pan, scraping the browned drippings into this water.
3. Pour this water (gravy base) into a small saucepan. Let the fat rise to the top; skim it off. Bring to a boil.
4. Mix 1/4 cup flour into 1/2 cup cold water.
5. Gradually add the flour and water mixture to the gravy base until the gravy reaches the desired thickness. Turn the heat down to low. Season with salt and pepper as desired.

Nutrition Information
15 calories per 1/4 cup; 120 calories per 2 cups
1/4 cup: 3g (90%) carbohydrate, less than 1g (10%) protein, trace of fat

Turkey Burgers
Yield
1 burger (4 ounces)

For non–beef eaters, ground turkey is a wonderful alternative to ground beef and is a good source of iron and zinc. Look for it in the poultry section or frozen food sections of larger grocery stores. These burgers are especially tasty with cranberry sauce.

**6 ounces ground turkey (yields about   Salt and pepper as desired
   4 ounces cooked)**

Optional: Add a drop of sesame oil to the skillet.

1. Shape the ground turkey into patties.
2. Cook over medium heat in a nonstick skillet.

Nutrition Information
225 calories per serving
One burger: trace of carbohydrate, 30g (55%) protein, 10g (45%) fat

Fish

If good health is your wish, get hooked on fish! The following tips will take the mystique out of fish cookery; fish is one of the easiest foods to prepare!

Buying Fish

Fresh fish, when properly handled, has no "fishy" odor either raw or cooked. The odor comes with aging and bacterial contamination. Whenever possible, ask to smell the fish you're wanting to buy. Signs of freshness to look for are bulging eyes, reddish gills, and shiny scales that adhere firmly to the skin. After buying fresh fish, use it quickly, preferably within a day. Keep it in the coldest part of the refrigerator.

When buying commercially frozen fish, be sure the box is firm and square, showing no sign of thawing and refreezing. To thaw, defrost in the refrigerator or microwave oven. Do not refreeze.

For each serving, allow 1 pound of whole fish (such as trout or mackerel) or 1/3 to 1/2 pound fish fillets or steaks (such as salmon, swordfish, halibut, or sole). To rid your hands of any fishy smell, rub them with lemon juice or vinegar. Wash cooking utensils with 1 teaspoon baking soda per quart of water.

Cooking Tips

Here are a few tips to help you prepare your "catch."

- If possible, cook fish in its serving dish; fish is fragile and more attractive the less it is handled.
- Seasonings that go well with fish include lemon, dill, basil, rosemary, and parsley (and paprika, for color).
- To test for doneness, gently pull the flesh apart with a fork. It should flake easily and no longer be translucent.
- Use leftover fish, either warm or cold, in sandwiches as a change from chicken or turkey.

Broiling. Place fish on a broiling pan that has been lightly oiled to prevent sticking, sprinkle with a little olive oil and seasonings (if desired), and place 4 to 6 inches from the heat source. Thin fillets (such as sole or bluefish) can be cooked in 5 minutes (without turning); thicker fillets (such as salmon or swordfish) may require about 5 or 6 minutes per side.

Baking. Set the fish in a lightly oiled baking dish, season as desired, cover, and bake at 400° for 15 to 20 minutes, depending on thickness.

Poaching. Cover fish fillets with water, white wine, or milk; season as desired and gently simmer for about 10 minutes.

Microwaving. If possible, place the thickest part of the fillet toward the outside of the dish, overlapping thin portions to prevent over-cooking. Season as desired, cover with waxed paper, and microwave for the minimum amount of time to prevent the fish from turning tough and dry. Remove the fish from the oven before it is totally cooked and allow it to stand for 5 minutes to finish cooking before serving. Whitefish fillets may need 4 minutes, salmon steaks 6 to 7 minutes.

Recipes
Broiled Fish Dijon

Crunchy Fish Fillets

Curried Tuna Salad

Fish and Broccoli Soup

Fish Florentine

Oriental Steamed Fish

Salmon Stew

Scallops Baked in Foil

See also: Baked Chicken With Mustard, Egg Drop Soup.

Broiled Fish Dijon

Yield
2 servings

Simple but tasty with that classic Dijon flavor.

1–2 tablespoons ''lite'' mayonnaise **1 pound fish fillets**
1–2 tablespoons dijon mustard

1. Combine the mayonnaise and mustard, and then spread the mixture on top of the fish.
2. Broil the fish 4 to 6 inches from the heat source for about 5 minutes or until it flakes easily with a fork.

Nutrition Information

200 calories per serving; 400 calories per recipe (made with cod)
One serving: trace of carbohydrate, 42g (85%) protein, 3g (15%) fat

Crunchy Fish Fillets

Yield
2 servings

Top with bran flakes or crushed shredded wheat for variety.

1 pound fish fillets

Salt and pepper as desired

2 teaspoons olive oil

1/3 cup Rice Krispies or cornflake crumbs

Optional: sprinkle with dried parsley flakes or parmesan cheese.

---

1. Preheat the oven to 450°.
2. Wash and dry the fish fillets. Cut into individual servings.
3. Season with salt and pepper as desired; coat with the oil.
4. Dip fillets into cereal crumbs; coat thoroughly.
5. Arrange the fillets on a lightly oiled baking dish and bake at 450° for 12 minutes; don't turn.

Nutrition Information

240 calories per serving; 480 calories per recipe (made with cod)
One serving: 8g (15%) carbohydrate, 40g (65%) protein, 5g (20%) fat

Curried Tuna Salad

Yield
2 servings

Tasty stuffed into a pita pocket. To reduce the fat content, replace part or all of the mayonnaise with plain yogurt.

2 tablespoons "lite" mayonnaise

1/4 teaspoon curry

1/2 8-ounce can pineapple tidbits, drained

1 7-ounce can tuna, drained and broken into chunks

Optional: 2 tablespoons chutney, chopped.

---

1. In a small bowl, combine the mayonnaise, curry, and pineapple (and the chutney, if you like).
2. Add the flaked tuna. If time permits, cover and chill the mixture to allow flavors to blend.
3. Serve on a bed of lettuce or in a sandwich.

Nutrition Information

220 calories per serving; 440 calories per recipe
One serving: 20g (35%) carbohydrate, 28g (50%) protein, 4g (15%) fat

Fish and Broccoli Soup

Yield
1 serving

Because fish cooks so quickly, it makes a simple soup in no time at all. I like this soup because it's simple to make, tasty, and low in calories. For a heartier meal, add rice or ramen noodles.

1 cup chicken broth (homemade, canned, or from a bouillon cube)

1 tablespoon cornstarch mixed in 1 tablespoon water

1/3 pound whitefish, cut into 1-inch cubes

1 cup fresh or frozen broccoli, chopped

Optional: 3/4 cup cooked rice or ramen noodles; 1/4 teaspoon sesame oil.

1. Heat the chicken broth. Stir in the cornstarch mixed with water to thicken the broth.
2. Add the cut-up fish and chopped broccoli along with the sesame oil, if desired. Bring to a boil, then turn down the heat.
3. Simmer for about 5 minutes or until the broccoli is tender-crisp and the fish is translucent.

Nutrition Information

200 calories per serving
One serving: 15g (30%) carbohydrate, 33g (65%) protein, 1g (5%) fat

Fish Florentine

Yield
2 servings

This goes nicely with rice or sesame noodles.

1 10-ounce box frozen chopped spinach

1/2 cup (2 ounces) shredded mozzarella cheese

1 pound fish fillets

Salt, pepper, and lemon juice as desired

1. Preheat the oven to 400°.
2. Thaw the spinach and squeeze out excess moisture. Layer on the bottom of a small baking dish.
3. Sprinkle with the cheese and top with the fish. Season as desired.
4. Cover with foil. Bake for 20 minutes or until the fish flakes easily.

Nutrition Information

280 calories per serving; 560 calories per recipe (made with cod)
One serving: 6g (10%) carbohydrates, 50g (70%) protein, 6g (20%) fat

Oriental Steamed Fish

Yield
2 servings

The scallions add a nice gentle flavor. If you have none, use onion instead.

1 teaspoon oil, preferably sesame

1 pound fresh fish

2 scallions, chopped

1 tablespoon soy sauce

2 tablespoons water

1. Heat oil in the bottom of a skillet.
2. Add the fish. Cover with the scallions and soy sauce. Add the water.
3. Cover and cook over low heat for 15 minutes or until the fish flakes easily.

Nutrition Information

210 calories per serving; 420 calories per recipe
One serving: 3g (5%) carbohydrate, 42g (80%) protein, 3g (15%) fat

Salmon Stew

Yield
3 servings

Salmon is among the best sources of fish-oil, the omega-3 fats that protect against heart disease. Eat if often, and enjoy your good health as well as a good meal! This stew goes nicely with corn bread or crackers.

1 15-ounce can stewed tomatoes

1 7-ounce can salmon, drained

1 12-ounce can corn

1 5-ounce can evaporated skim milk with 1 can water

Salt and pepper as desired

Optional: 1/2 teaspoon sugar, 1 teaspoon dill.

1. In a saucepan, heat the tomatoes, salmon, and corn (with liquid).
2. Add the evaporated milk, water, and seasonings as desired. Warm until heated; do not boil.

Nutrition Information
270 calories per serving; 810 calories per recipe
One serving: 37g (55%) carbohydrate, 10g (30%) protein, 4g (15%) fat

Scallops Baked in Foil

Yield
2 servings

Moist and tasty, this is an easily prepared "company dish" that leaves you with little cleanup.

Heavy-duty foil

4 cups vegetables, such as a combination of broccoli, bok choy, snow peas, sliced mushrooms, and water chestnuts

1 pound scallops

Salt and pepper as desired

1. Cut two sheets of foil, each about 18 inches square.
2. Cut the vegetables into bite-size pieces.
3. Mix together the vegetables, scallops, and seasonings as desired.
4. Divide the mixture onto the foil squares. For each square, bring two sides of the foil up over the food, fold together, and then fold the short ends towards the center, crimping to seal.
5. Place the foil packets on a baking sheet. Bake in a 450° oven for 20 minutes.
6. Place each package on a plate. (Do NOT try to lift them by the foil—use a spatula!)
7. Cut open the top to make a "bowl"; be careful not to burn yourself on the steam. Serve with rice.

Nutrition Information
280 calories per serving; 560 calories per recipe
One serving: 25g (35%) carbohydrate, 45g (65%) protein, trace of fat

Beef and Pork

Despite popular belief, lean beef and pork can be a part of a heart-healthy diet. They are excellent sources of protein, iron, and zinc—nutrients important for everyone, particularly athletes. The health problem with red meat is its fat content. To reduce fat, trim it off, choose lean cuts, and eat smaller portions.

For more information about low-fat meat cookery, refer to chapter 11 (Protein and Performance). For more information about iron and zinc, refer to the section on minerals in chapter 12.

Beef
Beef in Beer

Goulash

Hamburger-Noodle Feast

Stir-Fry Beef and Broccoli

Sweet 'N' Spicy Orange Beef

Tortilla Roll-Ups

See also: Chili, Tortilla Lasagna, Lazy Lasagna, Sloppy Joefus.

Pork
Pork Chops Baked With Apples and Sweet Potatoes

Pork Chops in Apple Cider

Stir-Fry Pork With Fruit

See also: Sweet and Sour Tofu, Low-Fat Fried Rice.

Beef in Beer

Yield
4 servings

This stew is a welcome winter meal. To save cooking time, use lean hamburger instead of stew beef.

1 pound extra-lean stew beef or top round, cut into small 1/2-inch cubes, or 1 pound of lean hamburger, browned and drained

2 large onions, sliced

4 large carrots, cut into 1-inch chunks

4 potatoes, quartered

2 12-ounce cans beer

1 tablespoon sugar

2 tablespoons vinegar

2–4 teaspoons salt or 2–4 bouillon cubes, as desired

pepper to taste

1. Brown the beef in the bottom of a large pot.
2. Add the vegetables, beer, and remaining ingredients.
3. Cover and cook over low heat for 1/2 hour. Add more beer or water as needed.
4. Skim the fat from the top.

Nutrition Information

400 calories per serving; 1,600 calories per recipe
One serving: 60g (60%) carbohydrate, 30g (30%) protein, 5g (10%) fat

Goulash

Yield
4 servings

The original recipe calls for stew beef, but I generally make this with lean hamburger to reduce the cooking time. Serve with noodles and peas to boost the carbohydrate content of the meal.

1 pound extra lean hamburger	**1 8-ounce can tomato sauce**
1 large onion, chopped	**1/8 teaspoon ground cloves**
1/2 teaspoon garlic powder or 1 clove garlic, minced	**1/2 teaspoon basil**
	Salt and pepper as desired

1. In a large skillet, brown the hamburger, onion, and garlic. Drain the grease.
2. Add the tomato sauce and seasonings. Cover and simmer for 20 minutes to 2 hours (longer time yields better flavor).

Nutrition Information

180 calories per serving; 720 calories per recipe
One serving: 10g (20%) carbohydrate, 25g (55%) protein, 5g (25%) fat

Hamburger-Noodle Feast

Yield
6 servings

When there's a potluck supper for members of the Greater Boston Track Club, Sandy and Andy Miller keep everyone well-fed with this simple casserole.

1 pound uncooked noodles	1 10-ounce box frozen corn
1 pound extra-lean hamburger	1 10-ounce box frozen peas
2 large onions, chopped	1/4 pound grated cheddar cheese,
1 24-ounce jar spaghetti sauce	preferably low-fat

Optional vegetables: green peppers, mushrooms, celery.

Optional seasonings: 1–2 teaspoons chili powder, 1/2 teaspoon cumin; 1 teaspoon oregano, 1/4 teaspoon garlic.

1. Cook the noodles according to package directions; drain them when they are slightly underdone because later they will be baked in the oven.
2. In a skillet, brown the hamburger and chopped onion. Drain the fat.
3. Add the spaghetti sauce and simmer for a few minutes to blend the flavors.
4. In a large casserole, combine the noodles, meat sauce, and still-frozen corn and peas; mix well.
5. Top with the grated cheese. Cover and bake at 350° for 30 minutes.

Nutrition Information
575 calories per serving; 3,440 calories per recipe
One serving: 80g (55%) carbohydrate, 43g (30%) protein, 10g (15%) fat

Stir-Fry Beef and Broccoli

Yield
4 servings

For a richer flavor, marinate the beef for an hour or overnight. Serve over rice.

1 pound extra-lean round steak or flank steak, thinly sliced	1/2 cup water
1 teaspoon oil	2 tablespoons soy sauce
1 pound (2 large stalks) broccoli, cut into flowerettes	2 teaspoons cornstarch mixed into 1 tablespoon water

Optional marinade: 2 tablespoons soy sauce and 1 tablespoon sherry.

Optional vegetables: sliced onions; mushrooms; carrots.

Optional seasonings: 1 teaspoon sesame oil; dash of hot pepper.

1. Slice the beef into thin strips. If time permits, place in marinade and refrigerate 1 hour or overnight.
2. Heat a large skillet, wok, or nonstick frying pan until very hot. Add 1 teaspoon oil, then the beef. Stir quickly, browning the beef on all sides. Remove the beef onto a serving platter.
3. Add the broccoli to the frying pan along with water and soy sauce. Cover and steam until tender-crisp, about 5 minutes.
4. Return the beef to the pan; stir in the cornstarch-water mixture; cook until the liquid reaches desired consistency.

Nutrition Information

210 calories per serving; 840 calories per recipe
One serving: 10g (20%) carbohydrate, 35g (65%) protein, 4g (15%) fat

Sweet 'N' Spicy Orange Beef

Yield
4 servings

Here's a welcome treat after a hard workout when you're hankering for something sweet but healthful.

1 cup uncooked rice   **1/4 cup orange marmalade**

1 pound extra-lean ground beef

Optional seasonings: 1/4 teaspoon red pepper flakes; few dashes cayenne pepper.

Optional mix-ins: cooked peas, diced celery, green peppers, pineapple chunks.

1. Cook the rice according to package directions.
2. In a skillet, cook the beef until browned; drain the fat.
3. To the beef, add the marmalade, hot pepper, and cooked rice. Mix well. Add mix-ins as desired.

Nutrition Information

375 calories per serving; 1,500 calories per recipe
One serving: 52g (55%) carbohydrate, 33g (35%) protein, 4g (10%) fat

Tortilla Roll-Ups

Yield
4 servings (1 1/2 tortillas each)

This quick and easy casserole is a popular "family food." You can also make it with ground turkey or diced chicken. For a vegetarian meal, replace the beef with kidney or pinto beans, and add chopped vegetables such as mushrooms, green peppers, and onions.

3/4 pound extra-lean ground beef

1 cup low-fat cottage cheese

1 tablespoon flour

1/2 teaspoon oregano

1/2 teaspoon basil

1/4 teaspoon garlic powder

Salt and pepper as desired

1 to 1 1/2 cups spaghetti sauce

6   6" tortillas

Optional: 4 ounces shredded mozzarella cheese.

---

1. In a skillet, cook the beef (or turkey) until browned; drain the fat.
2. Stir in the cottage cheese and flour. Add the seasonings as desired.
3. Put a thin layer of tomato sauce in the bottom of a 9" × 9" baking pan.
4. Spoon about 1/3 cup meat mixture onto each tortilla; roll up jelly roll style. Place the tortillas seam-down in the tomato sauce in the baking pan.
5. Pour the remaining sauce over the tortillas.
6. Cover with foil; bake in a 350° oven for 30 minutes.
7. If desired, uncover and sprinkle with mozzarella; bake for 3 minutes longer or until cheese melts.

Nutrition Information

375 calories per serving; 1,500 calories per recipe
One serving: 40g (40%) carbohydrate, 30g (35%) protein, 10g (25%) fat

Pork Chops Baked With Apples and Sweet Potatoes

Yield
1 serving

Open this foil packet carefully to avoid getting burned by the steam.

1 lean loin pork cutlet, trimmed (about 5 ounces)

1 medium sweet potato

1 small apple

Optional: 1 tablespoon raisins; dash of cinnamon; salt and pepper as desired.

1. Slice the sweet potato thinly. Quarter, core, and slice the apple into eighths.
2. On a large piece of foil, put sweet potato slices, a pork chop, and then apple slices. If desired, sprinkle with raisins, cinnamon, salt, and pepper.
3. Wrap well; bake at 350° for 40 minutes.

Nutrition Information

450 calories per serving
One serving: 55g (50%) carbohydrate, 34g (30%) protein, 10g (20%) fat

Pork Chops in Apple Cider

Yield
1 serving

Apples and pork are a tasty combination. For a simple dinner, cook some rice along with the pork, adding extra cider or water. Serve over rice.

**1 extra-lean pork chop or pork cutlet,   1/3 cup cider
trimmed (about 5 ounces, raw)**

Optional: 1/2 onion, sliced; 1 apple, sliced; salt, pepper, and basil as desired.

1. In a saucepan or small skillet, combine pork and cider, along with onion, apple, and seasonings as desired.
2. Cover and simmer over medium-low heat for 20 minutes.
3. If desired, skim fat from broth; thicken broth with 1 teaspoon cornstarch mixed with 1 tablespoon water.

Nutrition Information

250 calories per serving
One serving: 10g (15%) carbohydrate, 10g (50%) protein, 30g (35%) fat

Stir-Fry Pork With Fruit

Yield
4 servings

This is a popular family food that appeals to children and adults alike. Pineapple is a nice alternative or addition to the mandarin oranges.

1 teaspoon oil

1 pound boneless pork cutlets, trimmed and sliced into thin strips

1/2 cup water

1/4 cup vinegar

2 tablespoons molasses

2 tablespoons soy sauce

1 medium apple, diced

1/4 cup raisins

1 11-ounce can mandarin orange slices

1 tablespoon cornstarch mixed in 1 tablespoon water

Optional: pineapple chunks; green pepper chunks; 1/4 cup chopped walnuts.

1. Heat the oil in a large skillet or wok. Add the sliced pork and stir-fry until browned.
2. Add the water, vinegar, molasses, soy sauce, diced apple, raisins, and mandarin oranges; add the peppers and pineapple as desired.
3. Bring to a boil; cover and simmer for 5 minutes.
4. Thicken the broth by slowly adding the cornstarch-water mixture and cooking until thickened to desired consistency.
5. Sprinkle with chopped walnuts, if desired.

Nutrition Information

300 calories per serving; 1,200 calories per recipe
One serving: 30g (40%) carbohydrate, 25g (35%) protein, 8g (25%) fat

Eggs and Cheese

Eggs

Eggs are a controversial food, having both positive and negative nutritional features. On the positive side, they are an economical and highly nutritious source of protein. They are nutrient-dense, supplying lots of vitamins and minerals and all essential amino acids. They store well in the refrigerator, are easy to cook, and are handy for breakfast, lunch, or dinner.

On the negative side, egg *yolks* are loaded with cholesterol. One large egg yolk contains about 210 milligrams of cholesterol, compared to 30 milligrams in an ounce of cheese and 60 milligrams in a small serving of chicken. When cooking and baking, you can substitute two egg whites (with a trace of cholesterol) for one egg yolk in most recipes. Another way to reduce your intake is to save eggs for quick and easy dinners, instead of eating them for breakfast.

Cheese

Cheese also has positive and negative nutritional aspects. Cheese is a good source of protein, riboflavin, and calcium. It's economical and versatile, it keeps well, and it can be an enjoyable part of breakfast, lunch, dinner, snacks, and even desserts.

However, full-fat cheeses are high in saturated fat, sodium, and calories. Fortunately for our health, the food industry is now making several brands of low-fat cheeses. People on sodium-restricted diets should be aware that these low-fat versions tend to be higher in sodium than the original cheese, so they should seek out the low-sodium brands.

Cheese tastes best when eaten at room temperature, but it's easiest to grate, shred, or slice when cold or even partially frozen. I grate and freeze the odds and ends of cheese that accumulate in the refrigerator. They're ready and waiting whenever I want a quick handful to garnish a hot meal or add to a casserole.

Eggs
Egg Drop Soup
Egg-Stuffed Baked Potato
French Toast With Cheese

See also: Low-Fat Fried Rice.

Cheese
Easy Cheesy Noodles

Lazy Lasagna

Pizza Fondue

See also: Tortilla Roll-Ups, Cheesy Bean and Rice Casserole, Pasta and Veggies With Cheese, Stuffed Shells, Pasta Salad Parmesan, Meal-in-One Potato, Greek Stuffed Potato, Potato Snacks, Eggplant-Tofu Parmesan, Tortilla Crisps, and Moist Corn Bread.

Egg Drop Soup

Yield
1 serving

Easy to make and low in calories. I often add cooked rice or ramen noodles to boost the carbohydrates.

1 cup chicken broth (homemade, canned, or from bouillon cubes)

2 teaspoons cornstarch mixed with 2 tablespoons cold water

1 egg

Optional: dash of soy sauce, hot pepper, and/or sesame oil; spinach leaves; broccoli, thinly sliced; bean sprouts; Chinese cabbage, shredded; bok choy, chopped; scallions, chopped; rice, cooked; ramen noodles, cooked; tofu, chicken, turkey, or fish (leftovers, or precooked in broth).

1. Bring the broth to a boil.
2. Beat the egg slightly, adding soy sauce if desired.
3. Thicken the broth by slowly stirring in the cornstarch and water mixture.
4. Stir the boiling soup quickly. While it swirls, slowly add the beaten egg. Remove from the heat. Do not stir.
5. If desired, add vegetables. They will cook in the heat of the soup, remaining crunchy but becoming warmed.

Nutrition Information

125 calories per serving
One serving: 8g (25%) carbohydrate, 8g (25%) protein, 7g (50%) fat

Egg-Stuffed Baked Potato

Yield
1 serving

If you let the potato bake while you exercise, dinner will be ready when you are! Or, prepare it in a microwave oven. Note: One of these potatoes alone may not provide adequate calories for a dinner. Plan to supplement this meal with soup and/or salad, or eat two potatoes.

1 large (1/2 pound, 3 1/4") baking potato	**1 ounce shredded cheese, preferably low-fat**
1 egg	**Salt and pepper as desired**

Optional: 1–2 tablespoons milk.

1. Prick the potato in several places with a fork. Bake it in a 400° oven for an hour or until done; potato should be tender when pierced with a fork.
2. Cut an X on top of the baked potato. Fluff up the insides and make a well.
3. For moistness add 1 tablespoon milk.
4. Break the egg into the well. Top with cheese and salt and pepper as desired.
5. Return to the oven until the egg is cooked, about 10 minutes.

Nutrition Information

270 calories per serving
One serving: 34g (50%) carbohydrate, 17g (25%) protein, 8g (25%) fat

French Toast With Cheese

Yield
1 serving

This is quick and easy for brunch or dinner. When served with maple syrup, it's my favorite "recovery food" after a long Sunday run.

1 egg or 2 egg whites, beaten	**2 slices whole grain bread**
1/3 cup low-fat milk	**1–2 slices cheese, preferably low-fat**
Salt and pepper as desired	

Optional: Maple syrup; orange marmalade.

---

1. Beat the eggs and milk; add salt and pepper.
2. Over a medium setting, heat a nonstick skillet.
3. Soak the bread in the egg and milk mixture; place in skillet.
4. Cook over medium heat until golden, turning once.
5. ''Sandwich'' each cheese slice between the two slices of french toast before serving.
6. If desired, serve with maple syrup or marmalade.

Nutrition Information

375 calories per serving plain; 525 calories with 3 tablespoons syrup
One serving: 78g (60%) carbohydrate, 26g (20%) protein, 12g (20%) fat

Easy Cheesy Noodles

Yield
4 servings

Another family favorite, served as a main dish with a green vegetable and salad or as a side dish with chicken or fish. Different types of cheese— parmesan, low-fat cheddar, or Swiss—offer different flavors.

8 ounces dry egg noodles

1 tablespoon olive oil

6 ounces shredded cheese, prefer- ably low-fat

Optional: salt, pepper, garlic powder, Italian seasonings; parsley, diced tomatoes, steamed broccoli, peas, or other vegetables.

---

1. Cook the noodles according to package directions. Drain.
2. Mix in the oil, seasonings to taste, and shredded cheese.

Nutrition Information

325 calories per serving; 1,300 calories per recipe
One serving: 45g (56%) carbohydrate, 18g (22%) protein, 8g (22%) fat

Lazy Lasagna

This recipe eliminates one big step—precooking the noodles! The noodles cook during the baking process, absorbing the water added to the tomato sauce. This recipe may seem skimpy on the cheese compared to other lasagnas, but it's designed for people who want to carbo-load, not fat-load.

1–2 10-ounce boxes frozen spinach or chopped broccoli

1 pound part-skim ricotta or low-fat cottage cheese or combination

1 tablespoon flour

1/4-1/2 cup water if needed to thin the cheese mixture

3 16-ounce jars spaghetti sauce diluted with 3 cups water

1 16-ounce box lasagna noodles

Optional: 4 ounces shredded low-fat mozzarella for topping.

Optional seasonings for cheese mixture: 2 teaspoons oregano; 1 teaspoon basil; 1/8 teaspoon garlic powder; salt and pepper.

Optional mix-ins: 1 pound browned hamburger, ground turkey, or chili beans; 1–2 cups sliced mushrooms, chopped onions, diced green peppers.

1. Cook the spinach or broccoli; drain.
2. In a large bowl, mix the vegetables with the ricotta, desired seasonings, and flour; add water if the mixture is too thick to spread easily.
3. In an oblong pan (9" × 13"), alternate 4 layers of the diluted sauce, uncooked lasagna noodles, and ricotta mixture, ending with sauce. Top with mozzarella cheese, if desired.
4. Cover tightly with foil and bake at 350° for 75 minutes. Let stand for 10 minutes before serving.

Nutrition Information

360 calories per serving; 3,600 calories per recipe
One serving: 55g (60%) carbohydrate, 14g (15%) protein, 12g (25%) fat

Pizza Fondue

This family favorite serves well as a friendly, informal meal. It's also ideal for camping trips or picnics if you have a small camp stove. To boost the carbohydrate content, eat more bread and less fondue.

1 16-ounce jar spaghetti or pizza sauce

8 ounces grated mozzarella cheese

2 tablespoons flour

1 loaf French or Italian bread, broken into chunks

Optional: celery chunks; green pepper cubes; mushroom caps.

---

1. Heat the spaghetti sauce in a fondue pot or medium-size saucepan.
2. Shake together the grated cheese and flour.
3. Gradually melt the cheese into the spaghetti sauce, stirring constantly.
4. Keep the fondue warm by placing the pot on a fondue-pot stand, heating tray, or camp stove.
5. Using forks, dip chunks of bread or raw veggies into the pizza fondue. Enjoy!

Nutrition Information

550 calories per serving; 2,200 calories per recipe
One serving: 77g (55%) carbohydrate, 27g (20%) protein, 15g (25%) fat

Tofu

Tofu, also known as bean curd, is made from an extract of soybeans. It is a complete protein that contains all the essential amino acids. Tofu has no cholesterol and is relatively low in calories and sodium. Surprisingly, about half the calories in tofu do come from fat—unsaturated fat, that is. Tofu is a popular alternative to meat, as well as a source of calcium for people allergic to milk.

Tofu is found in most supermarkets in the refrigerated vegetable or dairy sections. You can buy firm or soft tofu cakes that are packaged in water. To store tofu, drain off the water, place the tofu in a container with a tight lid, cover with fresh cold water, and keep in the refrigerator. If you change the water every other day, the tofu will keep up to 10 days without spoiling.

Tofu itself has very little flavor; it takes on the flavors of the foods with which it's prepared. For example, tofu mixed with soy sauce takes on a soy flavor; with chili, a chili flavor. It can be crumbled, sliced, or blenderized into a smooth cream. Due to this versatility, tofu lends itself to many recipes: spaghetti, salads, chili, Chinese stir-fry, and even salad dressings.

Recipes
Eggplant-Tofu Parmesan
Pan-Fried Tofu Slices
Scrambled Tofu
Sloppy Joefus
Sweet and Sour Tofu
Tofu Salad Dressing

See also: Chili, Stir-Fried Vegetables, and Egg Drop Soup.

Eggplant-Tofu Parmesan

Yield
4 servings

This dish tastes even better the second day, when the flavors have melded. It's a good sandwich filling when stuffed into a pita pocket. As a main dish, serve with rice. Lean hamburger or ground turkey can be used in place of, or in addition to, the tofu.

1 large (2-pound) eggplant, cut
 lengthwise into 1/2-inch slices
1 24-ounce jar spaghetti sauce

1 pound firm tofu, crumbled
1/2 cup grated parmesan cheese

1. Place the eggplant slices on a flat pan and broil for about 5 minutes on each side, until golden and tender.
2. Arrange half the slices in a flat baking dish coated with a thin layer of tomato sauce.
3. Add a layer of tofu, parmesan, and sauce.
4. Make another layer of eggplant, tofu, and sauce. End with a sprinkling of parmesan.
5. Bake covered at 350° for 25 minutes or until heated.

Nutrition Information

360 calories per serving; 1,440 calories per recipe
One serving: 27g (30%) carbohydrate, 27g (30%) protein, 16g (40%) fat

Pan-Fried Tofu Slices

Yield
1 serving

This pan-fried tofu can be eaten as a main course or in sandwiches.

1/3 cake firm tofu, sliced

1 teaspoon oil, preferably sesame, safflower, or canola

Seasonings as desired: salt, pepper, garlic powder, curry, cumin.

1. Slice the tofu into 1/4-inch–thick pieces. Season as desired.
2. Heat the oil in a skillet using a moderate setting. Add tofu.
3. Cook about 5 minutes per side, until golden and crispy.

Nutrition Information

200 calories per serving
One serving: 2g (5%) carbohydrate, 20g (40%) protein, 12g (55%) fat

Scrambled Tofu

Yield
4 servings

Scrambled tofu can be made in several ways, depending on your mood. Serve either with rice and vegetables or stuffed into a pita pocket.

2 teaspoons margarine or vegetable oil

1 small onion, diced

1 green pepper, diced

1 pound tofu, medium or firm, crumbled

Optional: raisins; chopped walnuts; sesame seeds

Optional seasonings: garlic powder; salt; pepper; curry or soy sauce.

1. Melt the margarine in a skillet; add the onion and green pepper. Sauté until tender.
2. Add the crumbled tofu and seasonings; heat thoroughly.

Nutrition Information

190 calories per serving; 750 calories per recipe
One serving: 5g (12%) carbohydrate, 18g (38%) protein, 10g (50%) fat

Sloppy Joefus

Yield
3 servings

This is a tasty version of the traditional Sloppy Joe.

1 bottle chili sauce

1 pound firm tofu, crumbled

3 bulky rolls or English muffins

Optional: grated low-fat mozzarella or cheddar-type cheese.

1. Pour the chili sauce into a saucepan.
2. Crumble the tofu into the chili sauce; heat over medium heat.
3. Toast the rolls or English muffins; top with the tofu mixture.
4. If desired, sprinkle with grated cheese.

Nutrition Information

445 calories per serving; 1,350 calories per recipe (without cheese)
One serving: 55g (50%) carbohydrate, 28g (25%) protein, 12g (25%) fat

Sweet and Sour Tofu

Yield
4 servings

This recipe is suitable for adding stir-fried chicken or pork. If it's too sweet or sour, use less sugar or vinegar. Serve with rice.

1 cup pineapple juice

1/4 cup soy sauce

1/4 cup honey or sugar

1/4 cup vinegar

1/4 cup catsup

2 tablespoons cornstarch mixed into
  2 tablespoons water

2 pounds firm tofu, sliced into
  1-inch cubes

2 green peppers, cut into strips

1 20-ounce can pineapple chunks

Optional: sliced carrots, celery, water chestnuts, other fruits or vegetables.

---

1. In saucepan, combine juice, soy sauce, honey, vinegar, and catsup. Bring to a boil, add the cornstarch and water mixture. Cook until thickened.
2. Stir in the tofu, green peppers, and pineapple chunks. Cook over low heat for 5 minutes.
3. Serve over rice.

Nutrition Information

500 calories per serving; 2,000 calories per recipe (excludes rice)
One serving: 13g (45%) carbohydrate, 30g (25%) protein, 17g (30%) fat

Tofu Salad Dressing

Yield
4 servings (1/2 cup each)

This is an excellent low-calorie way to boost the protein value of a tossed salad. Be creative with added seasonings—Italian, curry, Mexican, sweet and sour; whatever your favorite dressing, you can adapt it to this tofu base.

1 cake tofu (about 16 ounces)   Water and/or vinegar

Seasonings to taste: garlic, oregano, basil, and/or parsley; curry and sweetener; crumbled blue cheese; chili, cayenne, and/or cumin

---

1. In a blender, whip the tofu until smooth. Add the water and/or vinegar to make it the desired consistency.
2. Add seasonings to taste. Blend well. Store in a covered container.

Nutrition Information

140 calories per serving; 560 calories per recipe
One serving: 2g (5%) carbohydrate, 15g (45%) protein, 8g (50%) fat

Beans

Beans—protein-rich foods with little fat and no cholesterol—are one of nature's greatest foods. They can help lower blood cholesterol, control blood sugar, fight cancer, reduce problems with constipation, fuel muscles with their carbohydrates, and nourish muscles with lots of B vitamins, iron, zinc, magnesium, copper, and potassium.

Yet many athletes snicker at beans because of their potential to produce intestinal gas and discomfort. Beans can contribute to gas production because they contain types of fiber and sugar the body can't break down. Instead of being digested or absorbed in the small intestine like other foods, they pass into the large intestine where they're broken down by bacteria that are a normal part of the intestinal flora. There they ferment, forming carbon dioxide and other gases that can make you feel distended, crampy, or gassy. This flatulence is highly individual, depending on the bacteria that normally inhabit your large intestine. Some people can eat beans with no problems; other experience great physical and social distress!

Because beans are a healthful source of both protein and carbohydrate, vegetarian meals such as chili, hummus, bean-rice casseroles, and other bean-meals are perfect for a sports diet. When beans are the only protein source, be sure to combine them with complementary proteins, such as rice, to enhance their quality. (See chapter 11 for information about combining proteins.) Or eat beans with some form of animal protein, such as lean beef in chili or low-fat cheese on burritos.

The following recipes suggest some quick and easy ways to enjoy these high-protein, low-fat, carbohydrate-rich additions to your sports diet. Canned beans or home-cooked dried beans are nutritionally similar. I generally use the canned; they're quicker and more convenient.

For more complete information about preparing homemade beans and creating bean dishes, you might want to read cookbooks that specialize in vegetarian cookery. Appendix B lists some suggestions.

Recipes
Barbecue Bean Casserole
Beans Baked With Apples
Cheesy Bean and Rice Casserole

Chili

Hummus

Mexican Baked Chicken With Beans

Mexican Salad

Tortilla Lasagna

See also: Irish Tacos and Tortilla Roll-Ups.

Barbecue Bean Casserole

Yield
8 servings

Served hot in winter, these beans are a hearty side dish or entrée. In summer, I sprinkle them cold on a salad, along with a scoop of low-fat cottage cheese to boost the salad's protein value.

1 16-ounce can red kidney beans	3/4 cup barbecue sauce
1 16-ounce can pinto beans	2 tablespoons brown sugar
1 16-ounce can chick-peas	2 teaspoons mustard

1. Drain the beans.
2. In a saucepan or casserole, combine the beans, barbecue sauce, sugar, and mustard.
3. Simmer on the stove top over low heat for 15 to 60 minutes (longer time yields better flavor). Or, bake in a 350° oven for 30 to 60 minutes; uncover the last 15 minutes to thicken the sauce.

Nutrition Information

200 calories per serving; 1,600 calories per recipe
One serving: 35g (70%) carbohydrate, 10g (20%) protein, 2g (10%) fat

Beans Baked With Apples

Yield
3 servings

A simple variation on plain old canned beans. Add other fruits, such as raisins, pineapple, or pears, for variety.

1 16-ounce can baked beans	1 tablespoon mustard
1 tablespoon molasses	1 large apple, chopped
1 tablespoon vinegar	

1. Mix all the ingredients in a saucepan.
2. Simmer gently on the stove top for 10 to 15 minutes.

Nutrition Information

230 calories per serving; 690 calories per recipe
One serving: 45g (75%) carbohydrate, 10g (15%) protein, 3g (10%) fat

Cheesy Bean and Rice Casserole

Yield
4 servings

This is a hearty stick-to-your-ribs winter meal that's a welcome treat after skiing. Green chili peppers add a spicy zip!

3 cups cooked rice

1 16-ounce can kidney or pinto beans, drained

1 large onion, chopped

1 clove garlic, minced, or 1/8 teaspoon garlic powder

1 cup low-fat cottage cheese

1 tablespoon flour

3 ounces grated cheddar cheese, preferably low-fat

Optional: 1 4-ounce can green chili peppers, chopped.

1. In a large mixing bowl, combine the rice, beans, onion, garlic, cottage cheese, and flour (and chili peppers, if desired).
2. Pour the mixture into a casserole dish; top with the grated cheese.
3. Bake covered at 350° for 30 minutes.

Nutrition Information

400 calories per serving; 1,600 calories per recipe
One serving: 60g (60%) carbohydrate, 25g (25%) protein, 7g (15%) fat

Chili

Yield
4 servings

As with most casseroles, the flavor of chili improves with age. Make a big batch and enjoy it more as the week goes on! For variety, serve it as a Mexican Salad. Moist Corn Bread is a nice accompaniment.

1 large onion, chopped

1 pound lean hamburger

2 16-ounce cans kidney beans

1 16-ounce can crushed tomatoes

2 tablespoons chili powder

Optional seasonings: 2 teaspoons cumin; salt, pepper, and garlic powder to taste; 1 tablespoon molasses.

Optional mix-ins: chopped mushrooms, green peppers, broccoli, green beans; raisins.

Protein alternatives to beef: 1 pound diced tofu; 1 pound ground turkey; 1–2 cups corn; cheese shredded on top.

---

1. In a large skillet, brown the chopped onion with the hamburger or turkey. Drain the grease. If using tofu, sauté it with the onion in a little bit of olive oil.
2. Add the beans, tomatoes, seasonings, and optional mix-ins.
3. Cover. Simmer for 15 minutes to 2 hours—the longer, the better.

Nutrition Information

475 calories per serving; 1,900 calories per recipe
One serving: 30g (50%) carbohydrate, 47g (40%) protein, 5g (10%) fat

Hummus

Yield
8 servings (1/4 cup each)

This tasty, high-protein, high-carbohydrate spread is a wonderful alternative to peanut butter. You might find, as I did, that hummus becomes a favorite sandwich filling, snack (rolled into a tortilla), or dip for cucumber slices, green pepper strips, celery sticks, or pita wedges.

The secret ingredient in hummus is tahini—sesame paste. You can buy tahini in the ethnic food section of supermarkets or health food stores. Store leftover tahini in the refrigerator. Try tahini with pasta, too!

1 16-ounce can chick-peas

1 tablespoon lemon juice, bottled or fresh

1 clove garlic or 1/4 teaspoon garlic powder to taste

2 tablespoons tahini (sesame paste) or peanut butter

Salt and pepper as desired

Optional: dash of cayenne; 1 tablespoon parsley; 1/4 teaspoon cumin.

---

1. Drain the chick-peas, saving 1/4 cup of the liquid.
2. In a blender or food processor, mix the chick-peas, 1/4 cup liquid, lemon juice, garlic, tahini, and seasonings.
3. Blend until smooth. If you don't have a blender, mash the chick-peas with the back of a fork.
4. Serve with pita bread or as dip for vegetables.

Nutrition Information

80 calories per serving; 625 calories per recipe
One serving: 11g (55%) carbohydrate, 3g (15%) protein, 3g (30%) fat

Mexican Baked Chicken With Beans

Yield
4 servings

A spicy favorite! When cooking for myself, I wrap one piece of chicken with 1/2 can of beans in a piece of foil and bake it in the oven—no dishes to wash!

2 16-ounce cans pinto beans   **1 cup salsa**
4 pieces chicken, skinned

---

1. Drain the beans and put in the bottom of a baking dish.
2. Put the chicken on top; cover with the salsa.
3. Cover and bake in a 350° oven for 25 to 30 minutes. If desired, bake uncovered the last 10 minutes to thicken the pan juices.

Nutrition Information

350 calories per serving; 1,400 calories per recipe
One serving: 35g (40%) carbohydrate, 30g (35%) protein, 10g (25%) fat

Mexican Salad

Yield
1 serving

A cool, low-fat version of taco salad and an appealing summertime alternative to a bowl of steaming hot chili. I pack it into a plastic container for lunch at work, or enjoy it for a no-cook dinner.

1–2 cups chopped lettuce   **1 cup chili, cold (see recipe, p. 285)**

Optional: 1/2 tomato, chopped; 1 ounce shredded cheese, preferably low-fat cheddar; 1/4 onion, chopped; salsa to taste; Tortilla Crisps (see recipe, p. 298).

---

1. On a plate, put as much chopped lettuce as you'd like to eat.
2. Cover with the chili.
3. If desired, add optional ingredients (above).

Nutrition Information

325 calories per serving
One serving: 40g (50%) carbohydrate, 32g (40%) protein, 4g (10%) fat

Tortilla Lasagna

Yield
5 servings

Tortillas are an easy, precooked alternative to lasagna noodles, and they taste wonderful.

1 pound cottage cheese

1 1-pound can kidney or pinto beans

1 tablespoon flour

1/4 teaspoon dried red pepper or 1/8 teaspoon cayenne

Salt, pepper, and garlic powder as desired

1 tablespoon chili powder, as desired

6 tortillas, flour or corn

Sauce:

1 32-ounce can crushed tomatoes

2 tablespoons chili powder

1/4 teaspoon red pepper flakes

1 tablespoon molasses

Optional mix-ins: 1 10-ounce package frozen, chopped spinach or broccoli, cooked; 1 cup chopped vegetables; 1 cup corn; 1 pound lean ground beef or turkey, browned and drained.

---

1. Mix together the cottage cheese, beans, flour, seasonings, and vegetables as desired.
2. Make sauce by combining the tomatoes and seasonings.
3. Preheat oven to 375°.

4. In a 9″ × 9″ casserole, alternate layers of sauce, tortillas, and cheese mixture. Top with the sauce.
5. Bake, covered, 30 minutes. Let stand about 5 minutes before cutting into squares.

Nutrition Information

350 calories per serving; 1,750 calories per recipe
One serving: 22g (60%) carbohydrate, 22g (25%) protein, 6g (15%) fat

Beverages

Water always has been and always will be the ideal fluid replacement for thirsty athletes. When you tire of plain old water, try some of these liquid refreshers; they not only quench your thirst, but also refuel your muscles with carbohydrates and replace potassium and other nutrients that you might lose through sweating.

Recipes
Banana Frostie
Fruit Smoothie
Homemade Ginger Ale
Hot Spiced Tea Mix
Maple Graham Shake
Orange-Pineapple Delight
Strawberry Fizz

Banana Frostie

Yield
1 serving

A wonderful shake that tastes sinfully good! Whenever you have a surplus of bananas, peel them, cut them into chunks, and freeze them so they'll be ready and waiting to be whipped into this frosty treat.

1 banana, in frozen chunks　　　　**1 cup low-fat milk**

Optional: honey, brown sugar, or a sugar substitute; dash of cinnamon; 1/4 teaspoon vanilla.

1. Put the frozen banana chunks into a blender with milk.
2. Blend on medium speed until smooth.
3. If desired, add sweetener and flavorings.

Nutrition Information
230 calories per serving
One serving: 40g (70%) carbohydrate, 8g (15%) protein, 4g (15%) fat

Fruit Smoothie

Yield
1 serving

Fruit smoothies are popular for breakfast and snacks. The ingredients can vary according to individual tastes. Some tried-and-true combinations include banana and strawberries in orange juice and melon and pineapple in pineapple juice. Almost any combination works!

1/2 cup plain, low-fat yogurt   **1/2 cup fruit, fresh or canned**
1 cup fruit juice

Optional: substitute 1/2 cup low-fat milk or vanilla yogurt for plain yogurt; 1/4 cup milk powder, wheat germ, oat bran, or graham crackers.

1. Place all ingredients into a blender and whip until smooth.

Nutrition Information

250 calories per serving
One serving: 50g (80%) carbohydrate, 5g (10%) protein, 3g (10%) fat

Homemade Ginger Ale

Yield
4 servings (10 ounces each)

This has a delightfully refreshing taste—worth the preparation.

2 tablespoons fresh ginger root,   **1 cup boiling water**
  chopped   **1 quart seltzer**
2 lemon rinds
3–4 tablespoons honey, or other
  sweetener to taste

1. Put the ginger and lemon rinds in a small bowl with the honey.
2. Pour in 1 cup boiling water (or just enough to cover). Let steep for 5 minutes.
3. Strain and chill.
4. When ready to serve, add the seltzer water.

Nutrition Information

65 calories per serving; 260 calories per recipe
One serving: 16g (100%) carbohydrate

Hot Spiced Tea Mix

Yield
20 to 30 servings
(about 2 tablespoons of mix
per 6 ounces liquid)

This recipe, submitted by a member of the National Ski Patrol, is a welcome energizer on winter days. Its high sugar content quickly replaces the glycogen depleted by cold weather exercise.

1 cup instant 100% tea

2 cups sugar

2 cups Tang

1 cup lemonade powder mix (1 envelope)

1 teaspoon cinnamon

1 teaspoon cloves

1. Combine all ingredients, mix well, and store in a sealed container.
2. To prepare hot tea, add 2 level tablespoons of mix to 6 ounces hot water; most mugs hold 10 to 12 ounces.

Nutrition Information

90 calories per 2 tablespoons mix
One serving: 22g (100%) carbohydrate

Maple Graham Shake

Yield
1 serving

This is popular for a quick breakfast or snack. To make it into a higher calorie weight-gain supplement, add 1/4 cup milk powder and 2 or 3 more graham crackers. For variety, replace the graham crackers with breakfast cereals.

1 cup low-fat milk

1–2 tablespoons maple syrup

4 graham cracker sheets (8 squares), crumbled

Optional: dash cinnamon or nutmeg.

1. Combine all ingredients in a blender.
2. Cover and blend 1 minute on medium speed or until smooth.

Nutrition Information

400 calories per serving
One serving: 70g (70%) carbohydrate, 12g (10%) protein, 9g (20%) fat

Orange-Pineapple Delight

Yield
1 serving

A thirst-quenching way to boost potassium intake!

1/2 cup orange juice   **1 medium banana**
1/2 cup pineapple juice

Optional: 4 ice cubes or 1/4 seltzer, added to blender.

1. Combine the juices and banana in blender, along with ice cubes or seltzer, if desired.
2. Cover and blend at high speed until smooth and thick—about 1 minute.
3. Serve over ice.

Nutrition Information

240 calories per serving
One serving: 60g (96%) carbohydrate, trace of protein and fat

Strawberry Fizz

Yield
1 serving

Seltzer makes a wonderfully fun and foamy treat when added to blender drinks. Try lots of combinations—peaches, pineapple chunks, whatever!

1 cup vanilla yogurt (or low-fat milk)   **1/2 cup seltzer**
1/2 cup strawberries, fresh or frozen

1. Combine the yogurt and strawberries in blender.
2. Cover and mix well.
3. Add the seltzer; blend 2 or 3 seconds to briefly mix.
4. Pour into a tall glass. Be prepared for it to foam up.

Nutrition Information

210 calories per serving
One serving: 37g (70%) carbohydrate, 10g (20%) protein, 2g (10%) fat

Snacks and Sweets

Snacks and desserts are a major part of America's meal style. Fresh fruits are ideal choices in either case, yet there's a time and place for other sweets. The trick is to choose those lowest in fat and highest in carbohydrates. These recipes provide healthy alternatives to empty-calorie temptations.

Snacks
Cheesecake Snackwiches
Crunchy Peanut Butter Sandwich
Frozen Fruit Nuggets
Potato Snacks
Seasoned Popcorn
Tortilla Crisps

Desserts
Apple Brown Betty
Blueberry Buckle
Chocolate Lush
Zucchini Cake
A-to-Z Cake
Honey Carrot Cake
Oatmeal Raisin Cookies

See also: Granola, Banana Frostie, Honey Bran Muffins, Applesauce Raisin Bread, Banana Bread, and the other bread recipes.

Cheesecake Snackwiches

Yield
1 serving

In place of the graham crackers, try stone-ground wheat crackers, bagels, or English muffins. For variety, use cottage cheese instead of the cream cheese.

2 graham cracker squares   **1 teaspoon jam**
1 teaspoon lite cream cheese

Optional: sprinkling of cinnamon.

---

1. Spread one graham cracker with low-fat cream cheese.
2. Add the jam; sprinkle with cinnamon, if desired.
3. Top with the second graham cracker, making into a sandwich.

Nutrition Information

90 calories per serving
One serving: 16g (70%) carbohydrate, 2g (10%) protein, 2g (20%) fat

Crunchy Peanut Butter Sandwich   Yield
                                          1 sandwich

This sandwich is an excellent bedtime snack for people who want to boost their caloric intake. It can also be a satisfying breakfast, lunch, or dinner, but it's relatively high in fat (healthful fats, that is), so be sure to boost the carbohydrate content of the rest of the meal with fruit and juice.

2 tablespoons peanut butter   **2 tablespoons granola or sunflower**
2 slices hearty, whole grain bread   **seeds**

Optional: carbohydrates such as sliced banana, raisins, jam, honey, and maple syrup.

---

1. Spread the peanut butter on the bread.
2. Sprinkle on the granola and/or the sunflower seeds for added ''crunch.''
3. If desired, add jam, honey, maple syrup, raisins, or banana.

Nutrition Information

525 calories per sandwich
One sandwich: 45g (35%) carbohydrate , 17g (15%) protein, 30g (50%) fat

Frozen Fruit Nuggets

Popping a few of these frozen fruit chunks into your mouth is a refreshing treat after a hot summer workout. Frozen bananas are particularly good—similar to banana ice cream! These frozen chunks also whip up into delightful frosty shakes when blenderized with either milk or juice.

Grapes	**Watermelon**
Bananas	**Cantaloupe**
Strawberries	**Other fruits of your choice**

---

1. Cut the fruit into bite-size pieces.
2. Spread the fruit pieces on a flat pan and put in the freezer for 1 hour. When frozen, put the pieces into baggies, where they'll be ready for you to eat when the munchies strike!

Nutrition Information

50 calories per cup of nuggets
One serving: 12g (95%) carbohydrate, trace (5%) protein and fat

Potato Snacks

Yield
1 serving

Compared to restaurant-prepared potato skins, which are generally fried, this low-fat alternative fits better into a high-carbohydrate diet. When you are baking potatoes for dinner, cook a few extra to have on hand for snacking. Or pop one into the microwave oven.

1 large (1/2-pound) potato, baked	**Seasonings as desired, such as garlic**
1 ounce shredded cheese, preferably low-fat	**powder, chili powder, Italian seasonings, salt, and pepper**

---

1. Slice the potato into 1/2-inch coins.
2. Sprinkle with cheese and seasonings as desired.
3. Heat in the toaster oven or microwave until cheese is melted.

Nutrition Information

200 calories per serving
One serving: 35g (70%) carbohydrate, 10g (20%) protein, 2g (10%) fat

Seasoned Popcorn

Yield
1 serving (4 cups)

Popcorn makes a fun, low-calorie snack as long as it's prepared without lots of butter or oil.

Cooking Method	Calories per cup
Air-popped	25–40
Oil-popped	40–80
Oil-popped plus butter	75–100
Microwave bags	70–90
"Lite" brands	60–80

Popcorn "pops" because each kernel contains a small amount of moisture surrounded by a hard covering, the hull. When heated to 350°F (177°C), the water within the kernel turns to steam, which expands and bursts the kernel open, resulting in popped corn. One quarter cup of kernels yields about 7 or 8 cups popped corn.

If you don't have an air popper or a no-fat microwave popper, try this low-fat method for stove-top popcorn.

1 tablespoon oil, preferably safflower or canola   **2 tablespoons popcorn kernels**

1. Heat the oil in the bottom of a saucepan. Add the corn kernels.
2. When the popcorn is just about to start popping, carefully drain off half the oil but leave the kernels behind.
3. Resume cooking, allowing the corn to pop without the oil.

Season with: garlic powder or garlic salt; onion powder or onion salt; curry powder; oregano, basil, and/or other Italian seasonings; powdered salad dressing mixes; combination of red pepper and paprika; soy sauce; parmesan cheese or grated mozzarella; taco seasoning mix; cinnamon.

To get the seasonings to "stick" without butter, take some tips from some of my ingenious clients:

• Spray the popcorn with cooking spray, such as Pam, then sprinkle on the seasonings or buy seasoned popcorn sprays.
• Mix salt and water (or soy sauce) in a spray bottle, and "mist" the popcorn with the salt solution.
Note: People with high blood pressure should limit their intake of salted popcorn (see chapter 2).

Nutrition Information

150 calories per serving (with half of the oil drained)
One serving: 20g (55%) carbohydrate, 3g (5%) protein, 7g (40%) fat

Tortilla Crisps

Yield
1 serving

This low-fat version of nachos saves lots of calories yet offers an enjoyable "munch." Enjoy these crisps plain as low-fat crackers, or use them for dipping with salsa or refried beans. To make them into nachos, sprinkle the toasted crisps with low-fat cheese and chopped green chilies; heat in the oven for 5 minutes or until the cheese is melted.

1 6-inch tortilla: (white, whole wheat, or corn)

Seasonings as desired: garlic salt, chili powder, taco seasoning mix, grated cheese, and so on.

1. Cut the tortillas into chip-size wedges. Place on a baking sheet.
2. Sprinkle with seasonings to taste.
3. Toast in a 250° oven for 20 minutes or until golden.

Nutrition Information

50 calories per one small (6-inch) tortilla
One serving: 10g (80%) carbohydrate, 2g (15%) protein, trace (5%) fat

Apple Brown Betty

Yield
8 servings

This has always been a family favorite.

1/3 box (11 sheets) graham crackers	**3/4 cup brown sugar**
1/4 cup margarine, melted	**1 teaspoon cinnamon**
6 large apples, unpeeled	**1/2 cup water**

Optional: 1/4 teaspoon nutmeg, 1/4 teaspoon cloves; 2 tablespoons lemon juice; 1/2 cup raisins and/or chopped nuts.

1. Crush the graham crackers into crumbs by placing them in a plastic bag and rolling them with a rolling pin or a bottle.
2. In a bowl, combine crumbs with the melted margarine.
3. Put one third of the mixture in the bottom of a 2-quart casserole dish.
4. Core and slice the apples into thin wedges and put them into a bowl. Sprinkle the apple wedges with sugar, cinnamon, and other spices as desired.

5. Put the apple slices into the baking dish; add 1/2 cup water and then the rest of the graham cracker crumbs.
6. Cover and bake at 350° for 25 minutes; uncover, then bake another 15 minutes to crispen.

Nutrition Information

310 calories per serving; 2,500 calories per recipe
One serving: 58g (75%) carbohydrate, 1g (2%) protein, 8g (23%) fat

Blueberry Buckle

Yield
12 servings

There are few things that smell nicer than homebaked desserts! This cake is a favorite, not only for dessert but also as a coffee cake for Sunday brunch.

1/2 cup sugar

1/4 cup oil, preferably safflower or canola

1 egg or 2 egg whites

1/2 cup milk

1/2 teaspoon salt

2 teaspoons baking powder

2 cups flour, half whole wheat and half white

2 cups blueberries

Topping:

1/3 cup sugar

1/3 cup flour, preferably whole wheat

1 teaspoon cinnamon

2 tablespoons margarine

1. Preheat the oven to 375°.
2. Mix together the sugar, oil, and egg; add the milk, salt, and baking powder, and then the flour.
3. Fold in the blueberries.
4. Pour into a lightly oiled 8″ × 8″ baking pan.
5. Make the topping by combining the sugar, flour, and cinnamon and mashing in the margarine, using the back of a spoon. Crumble the topping over the batter.
6. Bake for 40 to 50 minutes or until a toothpick inserted near the center comes out clean.

Nutrition Information

215 calories per serving; 2,600 calories per recipe
One serving: 35g (65%) carbohydrate, 3g (5%) protein, 7g (30%) fat

Chocolate Lush

Yield
9 servings

This brownie pudding is a tasty treat for those who want a high-carbohydrate dessert after a wholesome meal. It forms its own sauce during baking.

1 cup flour

3/4 cup sugar

2 tablespoons unsweetened dry cocoa

2 teaspoons baking powder

1 teaspoon salt

1/2 cup milk

2 tablespoons oil, preferably safflower or canola

2 teaspoons vanilla

3/4 cup brown sugar

1/4 cup unsweetened dry cocoa

1 3/4 cups hot water

Optional: 1/2 cup chopped nuts.

1. Preheat the oven to 350°.
2. In medium bowl, stir together the flour, 3/4 cup sugar, 2 tablespoons cocoa, baking powder, and salt; add the milk, oil, and vanilla. Mix until smooth. Optional: Add nuts.
3. Pour into a lightly oiled 8″ × 8″ pan.
4. Combine the brown sugar, cocoa, and hot water. Pour this mixture on top of the batter in the pan.
5. Bake at 350° for 40 minutes or until lightly browned and bubbly.

Nutrition Information

230 calories per serving; 2,100 calories per recipe
One serving: 46g (80%) carbohydrate, 3g (5%) protein, 4g (15%) fat

Zucchini Cake

Yield
12 servings

This popular version of the A-to-Z Cake (see following recipe) is a tried-and-true favorite.

1 cup brown sugar

2 eggs or 4 egg whites

1/2 cup oil, preferably safflower or canola

2 teaspoons vanilla

2 teaspoons cinnamon

1 teaspoon salt

2 cups grated zucchini

2 teaspoons baking soda

1 teaspoon baking powder

2 cups flour, half whole wheat and half white

Optional: 1 cup raisins.

---

1. Preheat the oven to 350°.
2. Combine the sugar, eggs, oil, vanilla, cinnamon, and salt. Mix well.
3. Stir in the grated zucchini, then the baking soda, baking powder, and flour (and raisins). Blend gently.
4. Pour into a nonstick or wax-papered 9″ × 9″ baking pan. Bake for 40 to 45 minutes or until a toothpick inserted near the center comes out clean.

Nutrition Information

250 calories per serving; 3,000 calories per recipe
One serving: 35g (55%) carbohydrate, 3g (5%) protein, 11g (40%) fat

A-to-Z Cake

Yield
12 slices

This recipe allows you to customize your cake! Follow the steps listed in the precedings Zucchini Cake recipe. Replace the zucchini with your choice of 2 cups of any of these foods:

Apples, grated	**Pineapple, crushed and drained**
Applesauce	**Prunes, chopped (1 cup)**
Apricots, chopped	**Pumpkin, canned**
Bananas, mashed	**Raisins**
Carrots, grated	**Raspberries, fresh or frozen, drained**
Cherries, pitted and chopped	**Rhubarb, finely chopped**
Coconut, fresh ground	**Strawberries, fresh or frozen, drained**
Dates, finely chopped	**Sweet potato, coarsely grated**
Eggplant, ground	**Tapioca, cooked**
Figs, finely chopped	**Tomatoes (use only 1/2 cup sugar)**
Grapes, seedless	**Marmalade (omit the sugar)**
Honey (omit sugar)	**Mincemeat**
Lemons (use only 1/2 cup juice)	**Oranges, chopped**
Peaches, fresh or canned, chopped	**Yams, cooked and mashed**
Pears, chopped	**Yogurt, plain or flavored**

Honey Carrot Cake

Yield
9 servings

Most carrot cakes drip with oil and coconut, but this is a simplified, higher carbohydrate version. Using strained baby food saves you the effort of hand-grating the carrots.

1/2 cup honey

1 egg or 2 egg whites

1/3 cup oil, preferably safflower or canola

2 4.5-ounce jars strained carrot baby food

1 teaspoon cinnamon

1 teaspoon salt

1 teaspoon vanilla

1 teaspoon baking powder

1/2 teaspoon baking soda

1 1/2 cups flour, half whole wheat and half white

Optional: 1/8 teaspoon nutmeg; 1/2 cup each golden raisins, chopped walnuts or almonds, and crushed pineapple.

---

1. Preheat the oven to 350°.
2. Mix the honey, egg, oil, carrots, cinnamon, salt, and vanilla; beat well. Add nutmeg, if desired.
3. Add the baking powder, baking soda, and flour; then add the raisins, nuts, and pineapple as desired. Blend gently.
4. Pour into a nonstick or wax-papered 8" × 8" baking pan.
5. Bake for 40 to 45 minutes or until a toothpick inserted near the center comes out clean.

Nutrition Information

200 calories per serving; 1,800 calories per recipe
One serving: 30g (55%) carbohydrate, 3g (5%) protein, 9g (40%) fat

Oatmeal Raisin Cookies

**Yield
3 dozen**

*This recipe offers a low-fat alternative to the majority of cookies, which
are 40 to 60 percent fat. Due to their lower fat content, these cookies have
a soft, rather than crisp, texture.*

**1/2 cup oil, preferably safflower or
canola**

1 cup brown sugar

2 eggs or 4 egg whites

2 tablespoons milk

2 teaspoons vanilla

1 teaspoon cinnamon

1 teaspoon salt

1 teaspoon baking soda

1 1/2 cups uncooked oats

1 cup raisins

**1 1/2 cups flour, preferably half white
and half whole wheat**

Optional: 1 cup chopped nuts.

1. Preheat the oven to 375°.
2. Mix together the oil, sugar, eggs, milk, vanilla, cinnamon, and
   salt. Beat well.
3. Add the soda, oats, and raisins; mix well, then gently stir in
   the flour.
4. Drop by rounded teaspoons onto a lightly oiled baking sheet.
5. Bake for 8 to 10 minutes or until firm when lightly tapped with
   a finger.

Nutrition Information
95 calories per cookie
One cookie: 15g (65%) carbohydrate, 1g (5%) protein, 3g (30%) fat

Appendix A
Nutrition Tips for
Diabetic Athletes

A regular diet and exercise program is important for proper blood sugar control for diabetics. The following nutrition tips may help a diabetic better enjoy an active lifestyle.

For additional readings, see Appendix B.

1. Exercise regularly. It's best to do this at the same time each day, as this will help you determine and stabilize your insulin and food requirements. Consistency is very important for optimal blood sugar control.

2. Exercise with someone else. This person should know that you are diabetic and be aware of the signs of hypoglycemia (confusion, weakness, unconsciousness, convulsions). If your blood sugar plummets, you may become incoherent and you might stagger and fall; you want your companion to be aware of what's happening. Make sure that your exercise partner also knows what to do in an emergency.

3. Do not inject insulin into the muscles you will be exercising. Exercise would cause the insulin to be mobilized faster, and you might become hypoglycemic. You would also have less insulin available to you later in the day or evening.

4. The average diabetic in training should not change the insulin dosage for training but should eat more food. If you repeatedly become hypoglycemic during or after exercise (despite eating more food), you should talk to your doctor about reducing your insulin.

5. If you're going to be participating in a one-shot bout of high activity (such as an unexpected basketball game), you should eat food before and may want to reduce your insulin. Through experience, you'll learn about your body and what works best for you.

6.   To best determine your energy/insulin needs, you'll want to monitor your blood glucose during training (for instance, between quarters of a football game or between laps of swimming). You may also need to reestablish these needs when the weather changes from hot to cold.

7.   Always exercise after eating, when your blood sugar is on the rise. Do not start to exercise with low blood sugar. Eat a snack first.

8.   Always carry sugar in some form with you. (Hard candies are popular because they aren't messy.) Also carry change with you for a phone call or a vending machine.

9.   During long-term exercise, replace glucose supplies regularly. When swimming, you may want to pop out of the pool after 50 laps to drink a small can of orange juice; during a marathon, you'll need to eat sugar or snacks along the route.

10.   A diabetic has an impaired ability to store and mobilize carbohydrates in the right amounts at the right times. So you should not try to carbo-load. Instead, plan to eat extra calories during exercise.

11.   On a long day trip of, say, hiking or cycling, eat six small meals containing both carbohydrate and protein. Be overprepared with extra "emergency food," in case you get unexpectedly delayed. Explain to your friends beforehand that you are unwilling to share that food with them.

12.   Drink plenty of fluids before and during exercise, to prevent yourself from becoming dehydrated. You need more fluid if your urine is dark and sparse.

13.   Exercise has a lingering effect, so you should eat more than usual after exercising. Otherwise, you may become hypoglycemic that night or even the next day.

14.   Wear comfortable shoes to prevent blisters and feet problems.

15.   Guard against injuries, and be meticulous with any that may occur.

Appendix B
Nutrition Resources

This list of resources provides additional sources of information on many of the topics discussed in this book. A few are primarily for professionals, but most are appropriate for the general public. If you can't find the titles in your local library or bookstore, order them directly through the publishers. Many of the titles are also available through the following sources of reliable nutrition materials:

Gurze Eating Disorders Bookshelf Catalogue, Box 2238, Carlsbad, CA 92008 (619-434-7533).

Low-fat Lifeline, 52 Condolea Court, Lake Oswego, OR 97035 (503-636-1559).

Nutrition Counselling and Education Services, 11,111 Nall Street, Suite 204, Leawood, KS 66211 (913-782-8230).

Cancer
Call the Cancer Information Service (1-800-4-CANCER) and ask for their booklet *Diet, nutrition & cancer prevention: A guide to food choices,* prepared by the National Cancer Institute.
Lindsay, A. (1988). *The American Cancer Society cookbook.* New York: Hearst Books.

Calories
Netzer, C. (1987). *The complete book of food counts.* New York: Dell.
Pennington, J. (1989). *Food values of portions commonly used.* Philadelphia: JB Lippincott.

Diabetes
Berg, K. (1986). *Diabetic's guide to health and fitness: An authoritative approach to leading an active life.* Champaign, IL: Leisure Press.
Hess, M.A., & Middleton, K. (1988). *The art of cooking for the diabetic.* Chicago: Contemporary Books.

Eating Disorders

Brownell, K., & Foreyt, J. (Eds.) (1986). *Handbook of eating disorders: Physiology, psychology and treatment of obesity, anorexia and bulimia.* New York: Basic Books.

Roth, G. (1986). *Breaking free from compulsive eating.* New York: Bobbs-Merrill.

Seixas, J., & Youcha, G. (1986). *Children of alocholism: A survivor's manual.* New York: Crown.

Stein, P., & Unell, B. (1986). *Anorexia nervosa: Finding the lifeline.* CompCare.

Woititz, J. (1983). *Adult children of alcoholics.* Pompano Beach, FL: Health Communications.

Exercise Physiology

Costill, D. (1986). *Inside running: Basics of sports physiology.* Indianapolis, IN: Benchmark Press.

McArdle, W., Katch, F., & Katch, V. (1986). *Exercise physiology: Energy, nutrition and human performance* (2nd ed.). Philadelphia: Lea & Febiger.

Wilmore, J., & Costill, D. (1988). *Training for sport and activity: The physiological basis of the conditioning process.* Dubuque, IA: William C. Brown.

Wilmore, J. (1986). *Sensible fitness.* Champaign, IL: Leisure Press.

Fast Foods

For a poster that gives information on the calories, fat, and sodium in popular fast foods, send $3.95 to *Fast Food Eating Guide*, Center for Science in the Public Interest, 1501 16th St., NW, Washington, DC 20036.

Tribole, E. (1987). *Eating on the run.* Champaign, IL: Leisure Press.

Fiber

Anderson, J. (1986). *Dr. Anderson's life-saving diet.* Los Angeles: Price/Stern/Sloan.

Westland, P. (1983). *The high fiber cookbook.* New York: Arco.

General Nutrition

Brody, J. (1987). *Jane Brody's nutrition book.* New York: Bantam.

Brody, J. (1985). *Jane Brody's good food book: Living the high carbohydrate way.* New York: Bantam.

Connor, S., & Connor, W. (1986). *The new American diet.* New York: Simon and Schuster.

Heart Disease

American Heart Association. (1984). *American Heart Association cookbook.* New York: Ballantine Books.

Cooper, K. (1988). *Controlling cholesterol.* New York: Bantam.

Eating to lower your blood cholesterol (a booklet that focuses on cholesterol and heart disease and defines dietary goals, including lists of the different fats in many foods) is available at no cost from The National Cholesterol Education Program, National Heart, Lung and Blood Institute, C-200, Bethesda, MD 20892.

Hachfeld, L., & Eykyn, B. (1988). *Cooking a la heart.* 1952 Howard Drive, N. Mankato, MN 56001.

Piscatella, J. (1987). *Choices for a healthy heart.* NY: Workingman Press.

The cholesterol index clock (a poster that rank-orders foods according to saturated fat, cholesterol and fiber content) is available for $3 with a self-addressed, stamped envelope from Cholesterol Clock, 500 Company Store Road, LaCrosse, WI 54601.

The life saver fat and calorie guide (a handy poster that lists the fat and calories in over 200 foods) is available for $3.95 plus $.50 postage, from Center for Science in the Public Interest, 1501 16th St. NW, Washington, DC 20036.

Sports Nutrition

American Dietetic Association (1986). *Sports nutrition: A manual for professionals working with active people.* PO Box 10960, Chicago, IL 60610-0960.

Coleman, E. (1987). *Eating for endurance.* Palo Alto: Bull.

Williams, M. (1989). *Beyond training: How athletes enhance performance legally and illegally.* Champaign, IL: Leisure Press.

Williams, M. (1985). *Nutritional aspects of human physical and athletic performance.* Springfield: Charles C. Thomas.

Traveling

Ehret, C., & Scanlon, L. (1983). *Overcoming jetlag.* New York: Berkley Books.

Vegetarian Diets

Lappe, F. (1980). *Diet for a small planet.* New York: Ballantine Books.

Robertson, L., Flinders, C., & Godfrey, G. (1976). *Laurel's kitchen: A handbook for vegetarian cookery and nutrition.* New York: Bantam.

Robertson, L., Flinders, C., & Ruppenthal, B. (1986). *The new laurel's kitchen.* Berkeley, CA: Ten Speed Press.

Thomas, A. (1978). *Vegetarian Epicure, Book 2.* New York: Knopf.

Vitamins and Supplements

Griffith, H. (1988). *Complete guide to vitamins, minerals, & supplements.* Tucson: Fisher Books.

Hausman, P. (1987). *The right dose: How to take vitamins and minerals safely.* Emmaus, PA: Rodale Press.

Tyler, V.E. (1987). *The new honest herbal: A sensible guide to herbs and related remedies.* Philadelphia, PA: GF Stickley, Co.

Yetiv, J. (1986). *Popular nutritional practices: A scientific appraisal.* Toledo, OH: Popular Medicine Press.

Weight Control

Bennett, W., & Gurin, J. (1982). *The dieter's dilemma: Eating less and weighing more.* New York: Basic Books.

Brownell, K. (1988). *The LEARN program for weight control.* University of Pennsylvania Dept. of Psychology, 133 S. 36th St., Philadelphia, PA 09104.

Ferguson, J. (1988). *Habits not diets: The secret to lifetime weight control.* Palo Alto: Bull.

Wellness

Ardell, D. (1986). *High level wellness: An alternative to doctors, drugs and disease.* Berkeley, CA: Ten Speed Press.

Fish, H.T., Fish, R.B., & Golding, L.A. (1989). *Starting out well: A parent's approach to physical activity and nutrition.* Champaign, IL: Leisure Press.

Newsletters

Environmental Nutrition. 2112 Broadway, #200, New York, NY 10023-21420. Monthly newsletter that clarifies the latest nutrition controversies.

Mayo Clinic Nutrition Letter. Mayo Clinic, 200 First St. SW, Rochester, MN 55905. A monthly newsletter that provides standard nutrition advice.

Sportsmedicine Digest. PO Box 2160, Van Nuys, CA 91494. Monthly newsletter dedicated to the prevention and treatment of sports injuries; includes nutrition tips.

Sports Injury Forum. 850 Boylston St., Brookline, MA 02167. Monthly publication written by the staff of SportsMedicine Systems.

Sports Nutrition News. PO Box 986, Evanston, IL 60204. Bimonthly newsletter that reports the latest research in health and fitness.

Tufts Nutrition Newsletter. PO Box 50169, Boulder, CO 80321. Monthly newsletter that offers detailed coverage of current nutrition concerns.

University of California, Berkeley Wellness Newsletter. PO Box 359148, Palm Coast, FL 32035. Monthly newsletter that provides the latest information on nutrition, health, and fitness research.

Professional Journals

American Journal of Clinical Nutrition, 428 E. Preston St., Baltimore, MD 21202.

Journal of the American Dietetic Association, 216 W. Jackson, Chicago, IL 60606.

Journal of Applied Physiology, 9650 Rockville Pike, Bethesda, MD 20814.

Medicine and Science in Sports and Exercise, 401 W. Michigan St., Indianapolis, IN 46202.

Physician and Sports Medicine, 4530 West 77th, Minneapolis, MN 55435.

Appendix C
Associations

The following associations also provide nutrition information:

American Anorexia/Bulimia Association
133 Cedar Lane
Teaneck, NJ 07666
(201-836-1800)

American Cancer Association
90 Park Avenue
New York, NY 10016
(212-599-3600)

American Coaching Effectiveness Program
Human Kinetics Publishers
Box 5076
Champaign, IL 61820
(217-351-5076)

American College of Sports Medicine
PO Box 1440
Indianapolis, IN 46206-1440
(614-637-9200)

American Diabetes Association
1660 Duke Street
Alexandria, VA 22314
(703-549-1500)

American Dietetic Association
216 W. Jackson Blvd. #800
Chicago, IL 60606-6995
1-800-877-1600

American Heart Association
7320 Greenville Avenue
Dallas, TX 75231
(214-750-5300)

National Dairy Council (nutrition education materials)
6300 North River Road
Rosemont, IL 60018
(312-696-1020)

National Strength and Conditioning Association
PO Box 81410
Lincoln, NE 68501
(402-472-3000)

Women's Sports Foundation
342 Madison Avenue, Suite 728
New York, NY 10173
(212-972-9170)

References

Acheson, K., Schutz, Y., & Bessard, T. (1984). Nutritional influences on lipogenesis and thermogenesis after a carbohydrate meal. *American Journal of Physiology*, **246**, E62-70.

American Psychiatric Association. (1987). *Diagnostic and statistical manual of mental disorders* (rev. 3rd ed.). Washington, DC: Author.

Ardell, D. (1986). *High level wellness: An alternative to doctors, drugs and disease*. Berkeley, CA: Ten Speed Press.

Belko, A. (1987). Vitamins and exercise—an update. *Medicine and Science in Sports and Exercise*, **19**, S191-S196.

Bergstrom, J., Hermansen, L., & Hultman, E. (1967). Diet, muscle glycogen, and physical performance. *Acta Physiologica Scandinavica*, **71**, 140-150.

Brisman, J., & Siegal, M. (1984). Bulimia and alcoholism: Two sides of the same coin? *Journal of Substance Abuse Treatment*, **1**, 113-118.

Brouns, F., Saris, W., & Rehrer, N. (1987). Abdominal complaints and gastro-intestinal function during long lasting exercise. *International Journal of Sports Medicine*, **8**, 175-189.

Burckes-Miller, M., & Black, D. (1988). Male and female college athletes: Prevalence of anorexia nervosa and bulimia nervosa. *Athletic Training*, **23**, 137-140.

Clark, N., Nelson, M., & Evans, W. (1988). Nutrition education for elite women runners. *Physician and Sports Medicine*, **16**, 124-135.

Colins, G., Kotz, M., & Janesz, J. (1985). Alcoholism in the families of bulimic anorexics. *Cleveland Clinic Quarterly*, **52**, 65-67.

Costill, D. (1979). Scientific approach to running. *Track and Field News*.

Costill, D., Bowers, R., & Branam, G. (1971). Muscle glycogen utilization during prolonged exercise on successive days. *Journal of Applied Physiology*, **31**, 834-838.

Costill, D., Coyle, E., & Dalsky, G. (1977). Effect of plasma FFA and insulin on muscle glycogen usage during exercise. *Journal of Applied Physiology, 43*, 695-699.

Costill, D., Dalsky, G., & Fink, W. (1978). Effects of caffeine ingestion on metabolism and exercise performance. *Medicine and Science in Sports and Exercise, 10*, 155-158.

Costill, D., & Saltin, B. (1974). Factors limiting gastric emptying during rest and exercise. *Journal of Applied Physiology, 37*, 679-683.

Halberg, F. (1983). Chronobiology and nutrition. *Contemporary Nutrition, 8*(9).

Hargreaves, M., Costill, D., & Fink, W. (1987). Effect of pre-exercise carbohydrate feedings on endurance cycling performance. *Medicine and Science in Sports and Exercise, 19*, 33-36.

Ivy, J., Costill, D., & Fink, W. (1979). Influence of caffeine and carbohydrate feedings on endurance performance. *Medicine and Science in Sports and Exercise, 11*, 6-11.

Ivy, J. (1988). Muscle glycogen synthesis after exercise and effect of time of carbohydrate ingestion. *Journal of Applied Physiology, 64*, 1480-1485.

Katch, F., Clarkson, P., & Knoll, W. (1984). Preferential effects of abdominal exercise training on regional adipose cell size. *Research Quarterly for Exercise and Sport, 55*, 249.

Nelson, M., Fisher, E., & Catsos, P. (1986). Diet and bone status in amenorrheic runners. *American Journal of Clinical Nutrition, 43*, 910-916.

Nutrition update: Sodium. (1984). *Dairy Council Digest, 55*(6).

Phillips, P., Rolls, B., & Ledingham, J. (1984). Reduced thirst after water deprivation in healthy elderly men. *New England Journal of Medicine, 311*, 753-759.

Rosen, L., McKeag, D., Hough, D., & Curley, V. (1986). Pathogenic weight-control behavior in female athletes. *Physician and Sports Medicine, 14*, 79-86.

Sherman, W., Costill, D., Fink, W., & Miller, J. (1981). Effect of exercise-diet manipulation on muscle glycogen and its subsequent utilization during performance. *International Journal of Sports Medicine, 2*, 114-118.

Sims, E. (1976). Experimental obesity, dietary induced thermogenesis and their clinical implications. *Endocrinology and Metabolism Clinics of North America, 5*, 377-395.

Sims, E., & Danforth, E. (1987). Expenditure and storage of energy in man. *Journal of Clinical Investigation, 79*, 1-7.

Staff. (1988, August). Is it necessary to cut back on salt after all? *Tufts University Diet and Nutritional Letter, 6*(6).

Stewart, M., McDonald, J., & Levy, A. (1985). Vitamin/mineral supplement use: A telephone survey of adults in the United States. *Journal of the American Dietetic Association, 85*, 1585-1590.

Van Horn, L., Liu, K., & Parker, D. (1986). Serum lipid response to oat product intake with a fat modified diet. *Journal of the American Dietetic Association, 86*, 759-764.

Watson, R., & Leonard, T. (1986). Selenium and vitamins A, E, and C: Nutrients with cancer preventive properties. *Journal of the American Dietetic Association, 86*, 505-510.

Webb, P., & Annis, J. (1983). Adaptation to overeating in lean and overweight men and women. *Human Nutrition: Clinical Nutrition, 37c*, 117-131.

Weir, J., Noakes, T., & Myburgh, K. (1987). A high carbohydrate diet negates the metabolic effects of caffeine during exercise. *Medicine and Science in Sports and Exercise, 19*, 100-105.

Weinberger, M. (1988). Salt intake and blood pressure in humans. *Contemporary Nutrition, 13*(8).

Woititz, J. (1983). *Adult children of alcoholics.* Pompano Beach, FL: Health Communications.

Suggested Readings

Evans, W., & Hughes, V. (1985) Dietary carbohydrates and endurance exercise. *American Journal of Clinical Nutrition, 41*, 1146-1154.

Lemon, P. (1987). Protein and exercise: Update 1987. *Medicine and Science in Sports and Exercise, 19*, 5157.

Lukashi, H.C. (1987). Methods for assessment of human body composition. *American Journal of Clinical Nutrition, 46*, 537.

Williams, M. (1984). Vitamin and mineral supplements to athletes: Do they help? *Clinics in Sports Medicine, 3*, 623-637.

Wilmore, J. (1983). Body composition in sports and exercise: Directions for future research. *Medicine and Science in Sports and Exercise, 15*, 21-31.

See also: Appendix B, Nutrition Resources

Index

About the Author

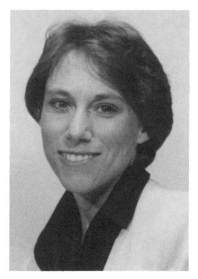

Nancy Clark

Nancy Clark, MS, RD, author of the highly acclaimed *The Athlete's Kitchen*, has been a dietary consultant to sport greats such as Olympic figure skater Kitty Carruthers, PGA golfer Brad Faxon, Wimbledon tennis player Tim Mayotte, and the Boston Celtics.

Nancy is a registered dietitian and the staff nutritionist for Boston's Sports-Medicine Brookline, one of the largest athletic injury clinics in New England, where she counsels casual exercisers and competitive athletes. She is an active member of the American Dietetic Association and its sports nutrition division, SCAN, as well as the American College of Sports Medicine.

A frequent speaker to sport and professional groups, Nancy also writes for *New England Runner, Runner's World, Bike Report*, and *The Physician and Sportsmedicine*. Boston area residents also know her through her weekly column in the *Boston Globe* sports section. An athlete herself, Nancy has biked across America, run marathons, and trekked in the Himalayas. She, her husband, John McGrath, and their son, John Michael, make their home in Waltham, Massachusetts.